Water Pollution & Health

Health and the Environment
Books in This Series

Water Pollution & Health

Cordelia Strange

AlphaHouse Publishing
New York

Health and the Environment
Water Pollution & Health

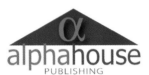

AlphaHouse Publishing
A Division of PEMG Publishing Group, Inc.
201 Harding Avenue
Vestal, New York 13850
www.alphahousepublishing.com

First Printing
9 8 7 6 5 4 3 2 1
ISBN: 978-1-934970-39-3
ISBN (set): 978-1-934970-34-8
    Library of Congress Control Number: 2008930667
Author: Strange, Cordelia

Cover design by Wendy Arakawa.
Interior design by MK Bassett-Harvey.

Printed in India by International Print-O-Pac Limited

 An ISO 9001 Company

Contents

Introduction

"The word *environment* does not mean something that surrounds us but an organism of all life within which we are fastened."
—Mose Richards, in
The Cousteau Almanac (1980)

Discussing the environment, we tend to speak as though it were a separate entity. "Protect the environment!" we demand, overlooking that *we* are an inseparable part of the environment. The air we breathe, the water we drink, the trash we discard, the sunlight to which we're exposed—all are different aspects of our environment. This series educates readers about humans' place in the environment and describes how intertwined our lives are with the natural world. Readers will also learn how certain human activities are degrading our environmental life-support systems, disrupting natural ecosystems and endangering human health in the process.

Among those at greatest risk for serious illness due to environmental pollution are children, the elderly, and those living in poverty, with children bearing the greatest share of the burden. According to the United Nations Environmental Program (UNEP), the quality of a child's environment is one of the key factors as to whether he or she will survive the first few years of life, particularly in developing countries. The World Health Organization (WHO) cites statistics showing that each year more than three million children under the age of five die due to environment-related diseases. Those claiming the highest toll include:

- Acute respiratory infections, 60% of which are related to environmental conditions.
- Diarrheal diseases, 80%-90% of which are a result of contaminated drinking water and poor sanitation.
- Malaria, the vast majority of cases resulting from lack of adequate mosquito control.

Such problems can only be solved through better environmental management programs. According to the WHO, preventing environmental disease could save the lives of as many as four million children each year. This series provides information on the health risks posed by environmental pollutants, describes ongoing prevention and management programs around the world, and offers useful advice to readers on how they can reduce their own risk of environmental disease.

Not only does this series describe how the quality of the environment affects us—it also explains how human activities affect the environment. Pollutants from automobile and factory emissions foul the air while wastewater from industrial discharges and inadequately treated sewage contaminate waterways. Improper disposal of hazardous materials and municipal solid waste can contaminate soils and groundwater, while careless use of chemical pesticides presents hazards to both humans and wildlife. Pollutants encountered in tobacco smoke, food, and water have been blamed for an increase in cancer rates and intestinal diseases. Humans create chemicals and wastes that foul the environment and these pollutants, in turn, can make humans sick. In addition, human population growth puts a steadily increasing strain on ecosystems, making environmental cleanup even more of a challenge.

Perhaps the greatest environmental threat of all is global warming. The predicted increase in violent weather, droughts, rising sea levels, spread of insect carriers of disease, crop failures, and resulting civil unrest will have a profoundly negative effect on people and the environment everywhere in the world.

We all need to learn how to make changes now to prevent irreparable damage to our atmosphere and our planet before it's too late. This series explores how the creation of new government policies and environmental laws is helping to bring about change and discusses how individuals can have a positive impact in their own homes and communities.

— Anne Nadakavukaren

Here's what you need to know

- Fresh water is essential to life on earth.
- Water has a liquid state, a solid state and a gaseous state.
- Water constantly moves through its three states as part of the water cycle.
- Urbanization alters the flow of water through the water cycle.
- Only 3 percent of the water on earth is fresh water.
- Poor water quality contributes to health problems worldwide.
- Direct pollution is known as point source pollution; indirect pollution is called non-point source pollution.

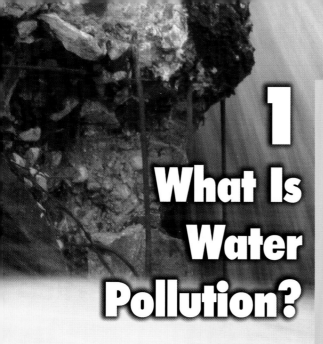

1
What Is Water Pollution?

Water, Water Everywhere…right?

Water is essential to our daily lives and important to the planet. Many people in the **developed world** use water everyday without thinking too much about it. People brush their teeth, water crops, shower, wash dishes, flush toilets, do laundry, and take the water for granted. This is a mistake. In fact, water is a limited resource that the world needs to be thinking about every day. In the **developing world** countries, poor water quality and lack of sanitation are major public health concerns. Around the world, urbanization, increased coastal development, and loss of wetlands are causing increased pollution in coastal waters. In addition, global warming and overuse of existing water resources are contributing to water scarcity concerns around the world. We need to learn how to save water, how to pollute our water less, and how to protect ourselves from existing water pollution before we run out of water and our Blue Planet becomes our Brown Planet.

Water's chemical formula is H2O. Because the two hydrogen atoms have a positive charge and the oxygen atom has a negative charge, water molecules are attracted to each other. This is why water has surface tension, and forms into drops.

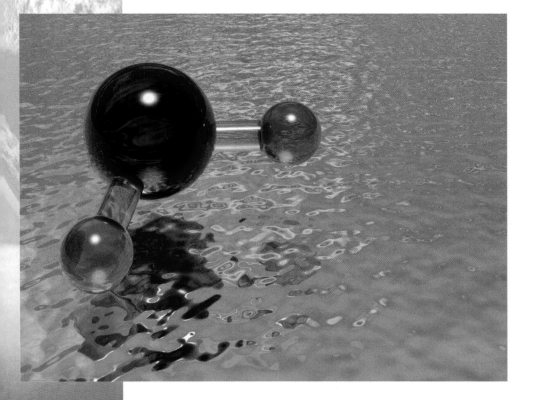

What is Water?

Some people think of water as the liquid that flows out of faucets or is dipped from a neighborhood well. Other people might picture ocean waves crashing against a beach, a still woodland lake, or a rushing river. Still others will imagine a gentle spring rain, fog rolling down mountains, or a harsh winter blizzard. A chemist will tell you that water is a molecule formed by the **covalent bonds** between two hydrogen atoms and an oxygen atom. Water is all of these things and more. Earth's water exists in many forms, or states, depending on where and when you "catch" it.

The Water Cycle

The amount of water on Earth always stays the same, but is constantly rotated through a system called the water cycle. The **colloquial** word "water" commonly refers to the liquid state of the substance, but water also has a solid state, ice, and a gaseous state, water vapor. The water cycle is a circle, so there is no beginning or end—and water can move either way in the cycle. Water vapor in the atmosphere one day could be liquid water in an ocean the next. If the ocean is then heated by the sun, the same water molecules could evaporate back into the atmosphere to turn back into water vapor. Precipitation occurs when enough water vapor collects in the atmosphere to form clouds. The water then falls from the clouds back to earth as rain, sleet, hail, or snow. Snow and ice store frozen water on high mountain peaks and in glaciers. Snow and ice can turn directly into water vapor through a process called sublimation. When snow melts it runs into streams, rivers, and lakes to replenish the fresh water storage supply on earth. This is how the water cycle has worked for billions of years, but times are changing.

Did You Know?

According the Environmental Protection Agency (EPA), a family of four in the United States of America can use as much as 400 gallons of water in one day alone. That is enough for one person to take 10 baths.

Did You Know?

About 55 percent of your body is made up of water. Almost 70 percent of the earth is covered in water.

Effect of Urbanization on the Water Cycle

The water cycle depends in part on the ability of precipitation to absorb through soil, be stored as ground water, and then slowly seep into streams and springs. However, in urbanized areas vast expanses of land are paved over with asphalt and concrete, which means that run off is unable to soak into the ground like it should. As a result, run off drainage patterns are altered. Streams are paved over to handle storm water run off from paved **impervious surfaces**. However, the extra water has nowhere to

Water Words

Condensation: the process in which water vapor is changed into liquid water.

Drinking Water: the water people use to drink, cook, and wash.

Evaporation: the process in which liquid water is changed into water vapor.

Fresh water: water that contains less than 1,000 milligrams per liter (mg/L) of dissolved solids; generally, more than 500 mg/L of dissolved solids is undesirable for drinking and many industrial uses.

Ground water: water stored underground

Precipitation: water released from clouds in the form of rain, freezing rain, sleet, snow, or hail.

Storm water: Storm water discharges are generated by precipitation and runoff from land, pavements, building rooftops and other surfaces.

Sublimation: the process in which ice or snow is changed into water vapor, without going through the liquid state.

Surface runoff: water from precipitation that flows over the surface of the ground downhill towards streams, rivers, and lakes.

Surface water: water visible on the surface of the earth in oceans, lakes, rivers, and streams.

Wastewater: Wastewater is the used water from homes, communities, farms and businesses that contains enough harmful material to damage the water's quality.

Water table: the top level of groundwater, below which the ground is always saturated with water, above it the ground varies from wet to dry depending on weather.

go, so there is an increased risk of flooding. There is also an increased risk of pollution as the water runs through sewers and over urban streets and parking lots.

Another effect of urbanization on the water cycle includes overuse of ground water drinking water resources. The use of too many large wells lowers the water table, causing other wells to go dry, pulling saltwater into drinking water wells, and sometimes resulting in sinkholes.

Fresh Water Storage

Fresh water storage is the most important part of the water cycle for life on earth. Without fresh water, humans and all living things on the planet would not be able to survive. Though it is vital to life as we know it, fresh water storage is only a small part of the water cycle itself—accounting for only 3 percent of all water on earth. 68.7 percent of the fresh water is held in glaciers and icecaps, 30.1 percent in ground water, and only 0.3 percent is held in sur-

Water is the only natural substance found in all three states—liquid, solid, and gas—at the temperatures normally found on Earth. Water freezes at 0°C (32°F) and boils at 100°C (212°F) (at sea level). Water is unusual because its solid form, ice, is actually less dense than its liquid form, which is why ice floats.

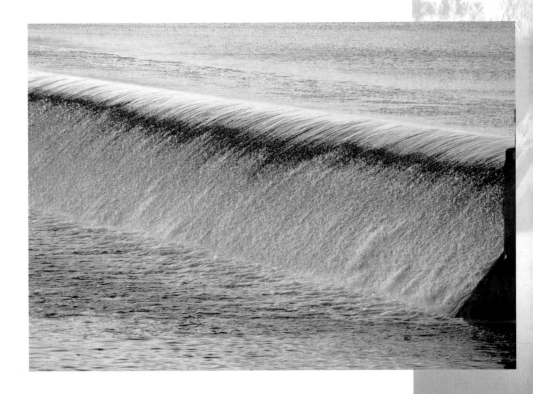

face water. This limited amount of water must meet the worldwide agricultural, industrial and personal demands for fresh water.

Agriculture is the largest consumer of fresh water, using 70 percent of the total worldwide fresh water supply, and up to 95 percent of the supply in developing countries. Industry uses about 21 percent of the water supply, and only 10 percent goes toward personal uses (hygiene and drinking). In addition, the distribution of water is uneven around the world, with some countries suffering more than others as a result of drought and flooding. Africa is the second driest continent in the world, in Ethiopia alone more than 57 million people have been affected by drought in the past 30 years. Ironically, flooding also causes water scarcity. In India, more than 70 percent of the annual rainfall happens during the three months of **monsoon**; often this water washes out to sea and farmers are still left with not enough water for their crops.

Water Pollution

The worldwide availability of fresh water is an important current issue, and with the global population increasing by two billion by 2030 the supply is only going to become more limited. However, water quantity is not the only issue; quality is also a major global concern. According to the World Health Organization (WHO), the quality of fresh water is important for drinking water, food production, and recreational water activities. Poor water quality contributes to heavy disease burdens around the world. Water contaminated with bacteria, viruses, protozoa and other microorganisms is a leading cause of infectious disease in both developing and developed countries worldwide. Certain diseases, like malaria, require water as part of the **vector**'s life cycle. In addition, improper sanitation and poor food hygiene contribute to water-borne diseases, especially diarrhea. According to the WHO, 88 percent of worldwide diarrheal disease can be attributed to unsafe water supplies, inadequate sanitation and poor hygiene.

Objects, chemicals and toxins that result from human activity can also affect water quality. This type of contamination is what is typically thought of as water pollution, and is defined by the United Nations Environmental Glossary as the presence in water of harmful or objectionable material from sewers, industry, or surface runoff. This harmful material affects the quality of the water, making it dangerous or unfit for human consumption. Water pollution also affects the health of natural ecosystems, such as wetlands, watersheds, lakes, rivers, coral reefs, oceans, and **estuaries**. Water pollution may come directly from a single source, called point source pollution, or indirectly from surface runoff, called non-point source pollution.

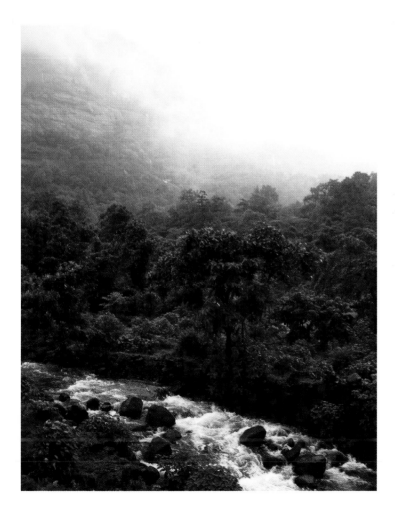

Water is called the "universal solvent" because it dissolves more substances than any other liquid. This means that wherever water flows, either through the ground or through our bodies, it carries valuable chemicals, minerals, and nutrients. This also means that it can dissolve and transport many negative substances.

Point Source Pollution

Point source pollution happens when harmful chemicals, toxic substances, or foreign objects are released directly into a body of water. This type of direct pollution includes pollution from individual, stationary locations such as factories, sewage treatment plants, and ships. Point source pollution may be the result of negligence or an accident, or it may be carefully regulated and planned. The 1989 Exxon Valdez Oil Spill is a prime example of accidental point source pollution. On March 24, the oil tanker Exxon Valdez traveling from Valdez, Alaska, to Los Angeles, California, ran aground of the Bligh Reef in Prince William Sound, Alaska. The tanker spilled 10.8 million gallons of crude oil, resulting in damage to the many fish, waterfowl, and marine mammals living in the sound. Waterfowl and marine mammals are especially hard hit if the oil covers their feathers or skin. The oil reduces **buoyancy**, and if

Water-based oil spills can cause extensive damage to aquatic ecosystems and the surrounding coasts. After the Exxon Valdez accident, oil covered 1200 miles of surrounding rocky beaches the clean-up began in April of 1989 and lasted until September of 1989.

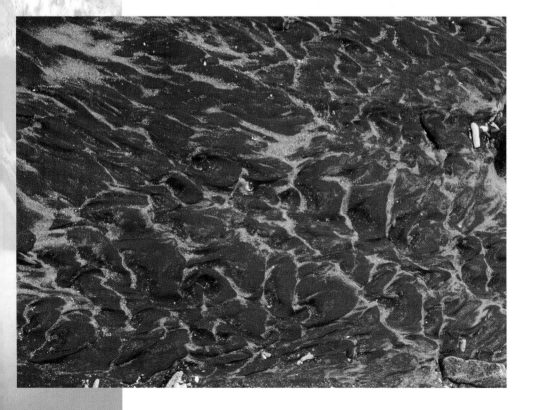

any is ingested during normal preening, or bathing, it can cause internal damage and probable death.

Chemicals in surface runoff from streets, parking lots, yards, and rooftops are major components of municipal pollution. In the United States, for example, as authorized by the Clean Water Act, the National Pollutant Discharge Elimination System (NPDES) permit program controls water pollution. Point sources include pipes and man-made ditches. Individual homes that are connected to a municipal system, use a septic system, or do not have a surface discharge do not need a permit; however, indus-trial, municipal, and other facilities must obtain permits if their discharges go directly to surface waters. Since its introduction in 1972, the NPDES permit program is responsible for significant improvements to the United States' water quality.

Most industrialized countries and many transitional countries have similar regulatory programs for control-ling point source pollution. However, according to the United Nations Environmental Program, regulations for the amount of pollutants allowed are often based on faulty assumptions or incomplete research. Hazardous water pollutants often include substances that are toxic, carcinogenic, **mutagenic**, or **teratogenic** at low concen-trations; these toxins can be **bioaccumulated**, especially when they remain in the water for long periods of time.

Human-made, solid objects floating in oceans, rivers, and streams are another obvious type of pollution. Known generally as marine debris, it is a problem along shorelines, in coastal waters, estuaries, and oceans around the world. Marine debris is any man-made, solid material that enters our waterways either directly or indirectly from a number of land-and ocean-based sources. Many humans live near the coasts, and the production of trash and the potential for marine debris continues to increase each year with the population. We need to control the disposal of trash and other wastes, or we will continue to find garbage in our rivers, streams, and oceans.

Non-Point Source Pollution

Non-point source pollution reaches bodies of water indirectly, via runoff that picks up and carries pollutants over or under the surface of the ground. These pollutants will be a combination of natural and man made chemicals and toxins that will combine in the run-off to be deposited in lakes, rivers, streams, wetlands, oceans, ground water, and drinking water. Pollutants may be broadly classified into categories including organic, inorganic, radioactive, and acidic or basic. The pollutants may include pesticides from farmlands, oil from urban areas, bacteria from livestock and septic systems, sediment from eroding construction

This image shows a wastewater canal in Oberhausen, Germany.

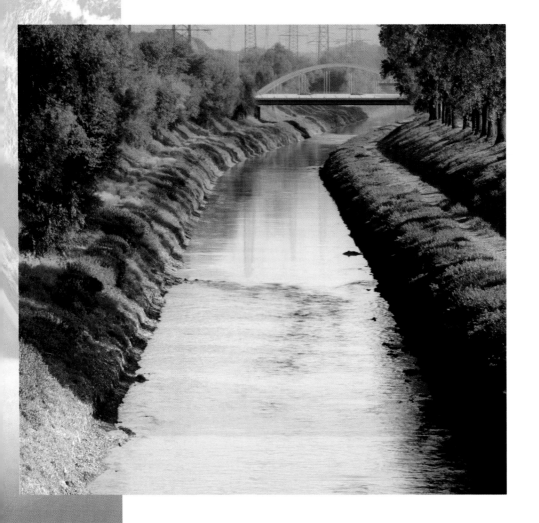

sites, and fallout from the atmosphere. Non-point source pollution is less obvious than point source, but the effects are in many cases more dangerous. Also, regulation of this type of pollution is more difficult because the sources are so spread out.

Sources of Non-Point Source Pollution

- Municipal: pollutants that flow from cities, communities, and homes. Sewage from treatment plants and chemicals in surface run off are the major factors in municipal pollution.

- Agricultural: pollutants that come from farms. Pesticides and nutrients are the major agricultural pollutants.

- Industrial: pollutants from factories. Metals, radioactive waste and other toxic chemicals are included in this category.

What are the effects of water pollution?

There are numerous effects of polluted water. Depending on the specific pollutant the effects include contaminated drinking water, unhealthy food animals (due to the bioaccumulation of toxins from the water), unbalanced marine and freshwater ecosystems that can no longer support biological diversity, and deforestation from acid rain. These direct results to water, resources, and ecosystems will then lead to indirect health and economic effects on individuals, communities, and the world.

STRAIGHT FROM THE SOURCE

From the UNESCO Water Portal Weekly Update No. 182, 30 March 2007

Lake Baikal is located in the south of Eastern Siberia, in the Buryat Autonomous Republic and the Region of Irkutsk, in the Russian Federation.

The territory of the Baikal watershed is extremely complex in terms of its political and administrative arrangements. Political borders split the Baikal watershed practically in half between Russia and Mongolia, although Lake Baikal itself lies entirely within Russia. Within the watershed there are 3 separate Russian states and 1 Autonomous Region; 12 Mongolian states; over 45 national parks; strict nature reserves and significant cultural sites in both regions; not to mention over 25 Russian and 116 Mongolian counties.

The lake covers 31,500 km2, is 636 km long, and 79.4 km wide at its widest point. Its average width is 48 km.

The Lake Baikal's water basin occupies about 557,000 km2 and contains about 23,000 km3 of water, that is, about 20% of the world's total unfrozen freshwater.

More than 300 rivers flow into Lake Baikal, the largest of them is the Selenga River which starts in Mongolia and provides over 60% of the lake's annual inflow. Only one river – Angara – flows out of the lake, it is called 'Daughter of Baikal'.

Lake Baikal is the deepest lake in the world. Its average depth is 730 m and its maximum depth is 1,620 m.

Being 25 million years old, it is the oldest lake in the world. It is known as the 'Galapagos of Russia', because its age and isolation have produced one of the world's richest and most unusual freshwater faunas. It is home to 1200 different species of animals, and 1000 species of plants. 80% of the species living in the lake are endemic.

In 1996 Lake Baikal was declared a World Heritage Site by UNESCO. The total area of the site is 8.8 million ha, of which 3.15 million are the lake's surface and 1.9 million are occupied by three reserves (Baikalsky, Zabaikalsky and Barguzinsky) and two national parks (Pribaikalsky and Tunkinsky). The Selenga River delta is protected by the RAMSAR Convention on wetlands because it is a key spot of North Asia in the flyway of migrant birds of the world.

The most famous and contested water pollution source in the basin is the Baikalsk Pulp and Paper Mill (BPPM). The factory is found on the southern shore of Lake Baikal and creates over 50,000 m3 of water pollution each year.

What Do You Think?

- Could the fact that Lake Baikal's watershed extends over two countries affect the protection of its water quality?

- What are some of the reasons UNESCO declared the lake a World Heritage Site?

- What do you think should be the responsibilities of the owners of the Baikalsk Pulp and Paper Mill in protecting Lake Baikal?

Find Out More

Water Cycle
http://ga.water.usgs.gov/edu/watercycle.html

Here's what you need to know

- A watershed is an area of land from which all run-off drains to the same location.
- Watersheds are important because all of our activities affect water quality at the end of the watershed.
- Precipitation and Infiltration are the two main factors affecting streamflow in a watershed.
- There are many other factors affecting water transit in a watershed.
- Sediment, nutrients, pesticides, and pathogens are pollutants that may be carried through a watershed.
- Pollutants cause environmental effects and health effects.
- Wetlands are important to the health of watershed systems.
- There are many types of wetlands all over the world; all are being lost to coastal development.
- An aquatic ecosystem is an interdependent group of organisms that live in a body of water.
- Aquatic ecosystems may be marine or freshwater.

Words to Understand

As **bioindicators** of water quality, fish are biological species used to monitor the health of a particular aquatic ecosystem.

Streamflow refers to the amount of water flowing in a river.

Chlorinated pesticides are carbon-based pesticides with chlorine atoms attached to them.

Atmospheric deposition occurs when pollutants are transferred from the air to the earth's surface.

Nearshore waters are the area extending seaward from the ocean shoreline beyond the breaker zone.

When a river overflows, the water spreads out over **floodplains**, which are flat areas of land that border the river.

When something is **adversely** affected, it is negatively changed.

An **invasive species** is one whose introduction and rapid spread through an area is negative

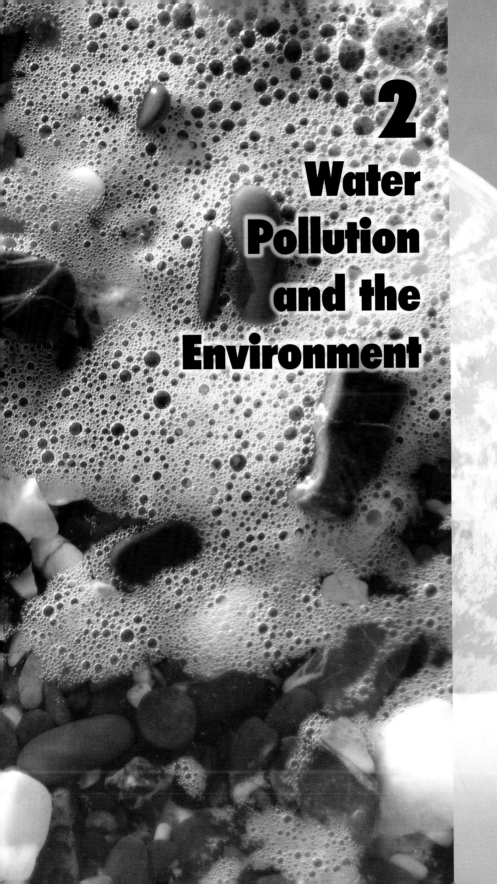

2
Water Pollution and the Environment

The most immediate effects of water pollution can be witnessed in the watersheds, wetlands, and aquatic eco-systems that become contaminated. Fish, waterfowl, plant life, marine mammals, and other life forms are often the first indicators of poor water pollution In fact, people are now looking to these life forms as **bioindicators** of water quality to let humans know whether water is safe for agricultural use, recreational use, or drinking water use.

What is a watershed?

When all the water on or under one area of land drains to the same location, that area of land is called a watershed. The watershed, also called a drainage basin or catchment area consists of all surface water and all ground water in an area. Every person on the planet lives within a watershed that drains to some larger body of water. A watershed can be a small valley with one lake at the bottom, or can encompass a large area and include all the lands and rivers that drain into an ocean. In fact, larger watersheds contain many smaller watersheds. Watersheds are important because the **streamflow** and the water quality of a river are affected by activity in the land area "upstream" from the outflow point.

What flows in does not always flow out

There are two main factors that determine how much water flows in a stream:

- Precipitation: The amount of precipitation that falls upstream as rain or snow is the greatest factor in determining rate of streamflow. However, a stream will often continue to flow even with no recent precipitation.
- Infiltration: After rainfall, some water soaks into, or infiltrates, the ground. Some water stays at the surface, where it gradually moves downhill, through the soil, and eventually seeps into the

stream bank. Some water travels deeper, and refills ground water aquifers.

Water may travel long distances or remain in storage for long periods before returning to the surface, depending on these factors:

- Soil characteristics: clayey or rocky soils absorb less water at a slower rate than sandy soils. Soils absorbing less water result in more runoff overland into streams.
- Soil saturation: Soil that is already saturated will not be able to absorb more water.
- Impervious surfaces: parking lots, roads, and developments rush rainwater right into storm drains that drain directly into streams.
- Slope: Rain falling on steeply-sloped land runs off more quickly than water falling on flat land.
- Amount of evaporation: The amount of evaporation depends on temperature, wind, and other factors.
- Amount of vegetation: Plants absorb water from the surrounding soil through their roots. Most of this water moves through the plant and escapes into the atmosphere through the leaves in a process called transpiration. Vegetation slows runoff, allowing infiltration.
- Reservoirs: Reservoirs increase the amount of water that evaporates and infiltrates. The storage and release of water in reservoirs can have an effect on the streamflow patterns of the river below the dam.
- Water use by people: The type of use and the number of people using the stream will affect the rate of change in streamflow.

Streams in a watershed vary based on all the factors listed above. However, during a strong storm, more water will flow in a few hours than flows normally in a few days.

A watershed is a system. A negative activity in one part of the watershed will affect another part, even hundreds of miles away. The following are some negative effects of watershed pollution:

- Pollutants such as sewage and marine debris can cause beach closings.
- Pollutants in bays and estuaries, as well as changes to the structure of the bay itself, can lead to loss of breeding and/or feeding grounds of fish, birds, and other aquatic animals.

This drain has evidently collected runoff from the farms surrounding it, and as such has collected heavy phosphorus and manure contamination. This organic richness has caused the algae bloom that we can see in the picture, covering the rocks where the water runs.

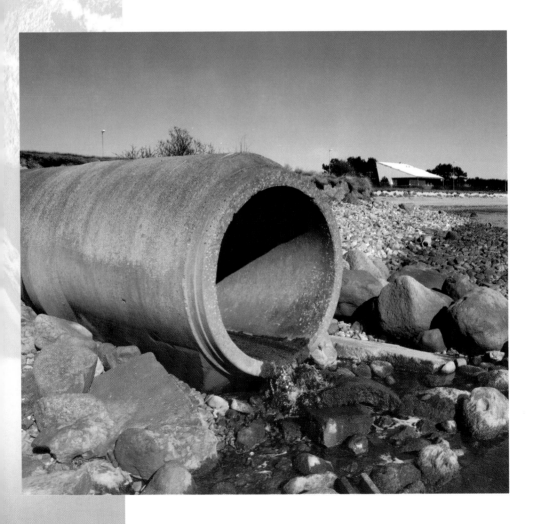

- Pollutants collect in **nearshore waters**, and affect aquatic ecosystems as well as causing loss of recreation areas.
- Marine debris and sediment carrying pollutants such as nutrients and pesticides can flow offshore and destroy coral reefs.

The Importance of Wetlands

Wetlands are areas where the ground is always saturated with water. Wetlands provide natural water quality improvement, flood protection, shoreline erosion control, opportunities for recreation and aesthetic appreciation, food resources and natural products for human use, as well as habitat for migratory birds and many of the world's threatened or endangered plant and animal species. Wetlands filter runoff before the runoff reaches open water. As the runoff water passes through, the wetlands retain excess nutrients, as well as some pollutants, and reduce sediments.

Wetlands are natural sponges that trap water and slowly release it. By doing so, wetlands act to slow the speed of flood waters and distribute them evenly over **floodplains**. This is especially important to have near urban areas where there is an increased rate of surface runoff.

According to the Ramsar Convention on Wetlands there are three major categories of wetland types, which are further divided into many other categories. Here is a sample of the divisions:

Marine/Coastal Wetlands

- Intertidal mud, sand or salt flats.
- Intertidal marshes; includes salt marshes, salt meadows, saltings, raised salt marshes; includes tidal brackish and freshwater marshes.
- Intertidal forested wetlands; includes mangrove swamps, nipah swamps and tidal freshwater swamp forests.

Did You Know?

If 1/2 inches of rain fall on 1/4 acre of land it would be equal to 3,394 gallons or roughly 85 baths!

• Coastal brackish/saline lagoons; brackish to saline lagoons with at least one relatively narrow connection to the sea.

Inland Wetlands

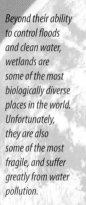

Beyond their ability to control floods and clean water, wetlands are some of the most biologically diverse places in the world. Unfortunately, they are also some of the most fragile, and suffer greatly from water pollution.

• Seasonal/intermittent saline/brackish/alkaline marshes/pools.
• Permanent freshwater marshes/pools; ponds, marshes and swamps on inorganic soils; with emergent vegetation water-logged for at least most of the growing season.
• Shrub-dominated wetlands; shrub swamps, shrub-dominated freshwater marshes, shrub carr, alder thicket on inorganic soils.
• Freshwater, tree-dominated wetlands; includes freshwater swamp forests, seasonally flooded forests, wooded swamps on inorganic soils.

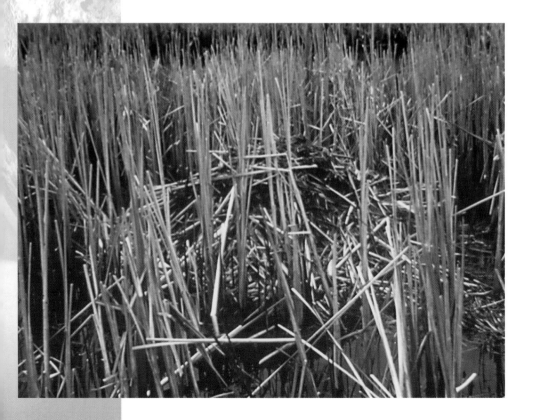

Human-made wetlands

- Aquaculture (for example, fish/shrimp) ponds
- Ponds; includes farm ponds, stock ponds, small tanks
- Water storage areas; reservoirs/barrages/dams/impoundments
- Excavations; gravel/brick/clay pits; borrow pits, mining pools.
- Wastewater treatment areas; sewage farms, settling ponds, oxidation basins

These wetlands are found all over the world and form a transitional space between the land and water; and between the terrestrial and aquatic ecosystems. When land-based pollution alters the quality of water flowing through the wetlands, or the wetlands are not there to filter the water, other aquatic ecosystems, and the humans dependent on them, suffer. Unfortunately, many of these vital wetlands are being replaced as a result of and increase in coastal development around the world. According to the United Nations Environmental Programme (UNEP), development on the coasts is projected to impact 91 percent of all inhabited coasts by 2050 and will contribute to more than 80 percent of all marine pollution.

What is an Aquatic Ecosystem?

An aquatic ecosystem is a group of interacting organisms that depend on each other and their environment for food and shelter. Aquatic ecosystems include any area in which water is a major component of life, such as wetlands, estuaries, and even floodplains. Aquatic ecosystems can be broadly divided into marine and freshwater categories. Freshwater ecosystems include reservoirs, lakes, rivers, streams, ponds, wetlands, as well as groundwater. Freshwater ecosystems are vital as sources of drinking water. Marine ecosystems are the oceans, coral reefs, estuaries, mangrove swamps, coastal systems, and intertidal areas.

Did You Know?

Even a single drop of water can be considered an aquatic ecosystem, as long as there are organisms living in it!

Besides the various and important services that marine ecosystems provide for the planet, they yield abundant food and economic benefits for people.

Water Pollution and Aquatic Ecosystems

Both freshwater and marine ecosystems are **adversely** affected by water pollution. Freshwater ecosystems are primarily affected by agricultural and urban runoff. Many freshwater plant and animal species are threatened or endangered because of human activity, pollution, or **invasive species**. Because the quality of freshwater resources is important to people, scientists have begun to use aquatic organisms as bioindicators of water quality. The scientists survey the health of the organisms, but they mainly consider the aquatic biodiversity of the ecosystem. Aquatic biodiversity refers to the variety of life forms within the ecosystem—a healthy ecosystem should have a good variety and the correct balance between predator and prey for that particular area. Both people and aquatic species benefit if pollution problems are caught early—a source of clean drinking water remains available, and biodiversity is preserved.

Marine ecosystems are contaminated by marine debris dumped into coastal waters, but are also heavily affected by pollutants carried via runoff. Most of this runoff enters at the outflow points of watersheds. Each type of pollutant is a concern for different reasons, but all have implications for loss of aquatic biodiversity, as well as effects on health and economic resources.

Types of Marine Ecosystem Pollutants

Sediment

One of the effects of increased urban and coastal development is increased flooding due to larger impervious areas. With increased flooding comes increased erosion as the power of the rushing water washes away sediment from construction sites, roads, farms, and other areas where dirt is exposed. When the soils wash into streams and rivers during storms and flow into lakes and oceans, the result is muddy water that reduces oxygen for animals living on the bottom, decreases the amount of light reaching plant life, and clogs fish gills. According to the Food and Agriculture Organization of the United Nations, sediment is also a major destroyer of coral reefs worldwide.

In addition to the physical damage caused by sediment, some kinds of pollutants bind to these sediments and flow into coastal waters. Phosphorus, **chlorinated pesticides**, and many metals are especially likely to bind with different sediments.

Nutrients

Excess nutrients, such as nitrogen, can also run off the land with rain and end up in coastal waters. Sources of nutrients include:

- fertilizers,
- pet and farm animal waste,
- decaying plants,

Did You Know?

Algal blooms are not a new phenomenon–Captain Cook recorded an algal bloom during his voyage in 1770. However, the blooms are becoming more frequent today because of increased ocean temperatures and higher nutrient levels that make for perfect algae growing conditions.

Bioaccumulation

Organic chemicals, such as pesticides and methylmercury that hitch a ride into the ocean with sediment particles, are of special concern because many of these contaminants are persistent, meaning they remain concentrated in the ecosystem, rather than dissipating over time. In addition, they enter the food chain at the lowest level and increase at each higher level of the food chain. The predatory fish at the top maintain high levels of the toxins. Which fish do we want to eat? The predators. Tuna are well-known for bioaccumulation of methylmercury. Eating tuna contaminated with mercury can cause neurogical damage, especially in children, whose central nervous systems are still developing. Therefore, children and pregnant women are advised not to eat tuna.

Did You Know?

More than 80 percent of marine pollution comes from land-based sources.

• failing septic systems,
• **atmospheric deposition**,
• poorly working sewage treatment plants.

In a healthy watershed ecosystem, nutrients in run off are processed by wetlands, which act as natural filters. However, the loss of wetlands has lowered the ability of watersheds to remove the nutrients from the water before they enter rivers, streams, and ultimately the oceans. In a process known as eutrophication, these nutrients cause algal blooms, blocking the light from penetrating the water. When the algae die, the process of decomposition uses up oxygen, leaving very little for fish and other aquatic life . In addition, some of these algae and related organisms release toxins that can kill organisms, and can be dangerous, sometimes even fatal, to humans.

Pathogens

Pathogens may also contaminate watershed systems. Pathogens are microscopic disease-carrying organisms like bacteria and viruses. They may come from untreated or inadequately treated wastewater. In fact, untreated wastewater discharged into the world's oceans is a serious threat to coral reefs, fishing grounds, and human health. According to UNEP, about 80-90 percent of the waste

In the Dead Zone

Dead zones are areas of the ocean that have very low-to no oxygen content. These hypoxic zones are caused by algal blooms that use up all the oxygen as part of their decay process. No oxygen means no life. Many fish are able to evacuate quickly, but shellfish, slow moving crustaceans, corals and other stationary organisms are doomed to suffocate. Most dead zones occur in coastal waters in areas that are also important fishing grounds. Some of these zones are natural in origin. However, between 2003 and 2006, the worldwide number of dead zones increased from 149 to over 200, which indicates that the increase in human activity on the coasts is related to the increase in dead zones.

water discharged from large parts of Africa and the Indo-Pacific is untreated. Pathogens in the water in unsafe amounts result in beach closures, shellfish bed closures, fish kills, and human health problems.

Other Pollutants

Pollutants, such as pesticides from farms and lawns and oils and greases deposited on roads from cars and trucks, all run off the land. Factories and sewage treatment plants also contribute to the amount of pollutants entering watersheds. Increased ocean acidification is also a major concern for marine ecosystems worldwide. As CO_2 in the atmosphere increases, the oceans become more acidic resulting in the loss of cold-water coral reefs and other organisms at the bottom of the food chain.

Ask the Doctor

Q: Tuna salad is my favorite lunch food, but my friends told me that it is like eating poison now and I shouldn't eat it anymore. Do I really have to give up my favorite food?

Your friends are referring to the fact that tuna is one of the fish that are known to accumulate mercury in their tissues. Mercury can cause brain damage if too much is taken into the body. You should try to keep to only 1-2 servings of tuna per week and if possible, use the canned light tuna, which is supposed to have less mercury on average than the albacore.

STRAIGHT FROM THE SOURCE

From the FAO document, Environmental emergencies affecting fisheries

Three types of environmental uncertainties affect fisheries:

1. natural environmental oscillations,

2. global environmental change, and

3. environmental emergencies.

Natural oscillations affect fish abundance and availability: seasonal oscillations are usually forecasted with reasonable accuracy and exploited by fishing industries whereas inter-annual oscillations that occur with a range of frequencies (such as 11 to 50-60 year cycles) are less predictable and are only slowly being understood (e.g. El Niño and La Niña phenomena).

Environmental emergencies correspond to environmental crises emerging as a consequence of an unforeseen combination of circumstances, such as the 2004 tsunami, with results that call for immediate action in the form of contingency plans or mitigating action, such as assistance or relief. These include fish kills, harmful algal blooms and oil spills (caused by tanker accidents or from incidents related to offshore development).

What Do You Think?

• How do natural environmental oscillations affect fish populations?

• How is global warming changing the natural environmental oscillations?

• What might this mean for fish populations?

Find Out More

Ramsar Convention on Wetlands
http://www.ramsar.org/ris/key_ris.htm#type

Vital Water Graphics
http://www.unep.org/dewa/assessments/ecosystems/water/vitalwater/

Here's what you need to know

- Urbanization has changed natural runoff patterns and has led to increased pollution of water sources.
- Hazardous chemicals and waste products contained in runoff enter surface and groundwater sources and seriously damage aquatic ecosystems and water quality.
- Storm water and associated flooding can overwhelm sewage treatment systems and spread polluted waters over large areas.
- Water sources can be protected by encouraging the natural environment around them.

Words to Understand

Snowmelt is runoff from melting snow

When something **subsides** it becomes less—it sinks or lowers

The **solid waste** of humans and animals is called feces.

A **levee** is a ridge or embankment built to keep a river or lake from overflowing

Evaporation occurs when a liquid (like water) turns into its gaseous (vapor) form.

To **saturate** is to soak, fill, or load to full capacity

An **aquifer** is an underground geological formation where the spaces between rock particles, sand, or gravel are completely filled with water. Water pumped from aquifers is referred to as "groundwater.

Persistent chemicals are those that remain in the environment for a very long time without degrading.

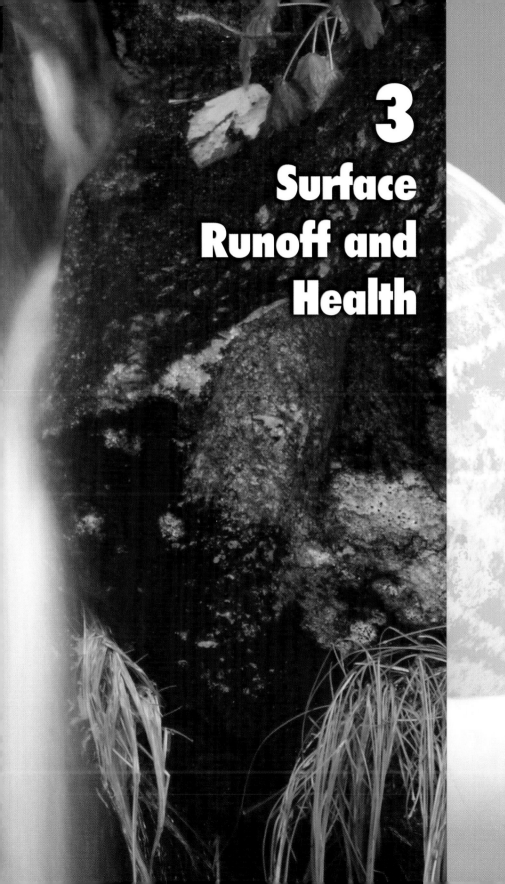

3
Surface Runoff and Health

Urban Runoff

Cities are sprouting up around the world. Even in countries that still rely heavily on agriculture, cities are growing. We call the process of moving people from rural areas into cities urbanization. Cities are characterized by high concentrations of people—lots of people in one place—and that means roadways, tall buildings, and sewage systems become necessary for a city run smoothly. Most cities develop near a source of fresh water. This can be an ocean or harbor, as in Mumbai, or it can be a large river, like in Paris, but either way, cities need fresh water just as much, if not more, than rural areas.

A city full of people creates a lot of waste, and the problem is keeping that waste out of the city's water source. All chemicals, garbage, and pollutants that enter a city's water source are categorized under "urban runoff." You see, unlike the varied terrain of natural landscapes, where grasslands and forests trap above ground waters, cities have mostly one type of landscape made of concrete, asphalt, and other impervious surfaces like rooftops. These surfaces do not allow rainwater and **snowmelt** to naturally return to the earth but instead channel them into unnaturally large collection points. When water is no longer flowing naturally, many changes can occur in the surrounding environment. Increased flow down sewers and drains can erode away riverbanks where drainpipes emerge, damaging streamside vegetation and wiping out aquatic life. Often urban runoff is a higher temperature than the water source it is entering, which can also harm aquatic life. If that isn't complicated enough, there is the additional concern that urbanized areas increase chances of flooding during and after heavy rainfall, as they channel rainwater quickly and at high speeds into nearby water sources.

But what has really gotten the attention of politicians and activists living in cities around the world are the pollutants urban runoff brings into our water sources. To better understand this process, let's imagine it from beginning to end: a storm moves in over a city like Chicago, Illinois. Rain falls onto the John Hancock building and slides down the sides of the 95-story building. Along the way, it picks up all the chemicals used to clean the building's many windows and then enters the sewer drains on the streets below. Before it enters the sewers, however, it picks up all the oils, grease, and toxic chemicals from cars and trucks, as well as any road salts or heavy metals left around. What we have now is potentially very toxic water moving very quickly along the impervious concrete lining of the sewer system. When it enters nearby Lake Michigan later that day, most Chicagoans will have no idea what sorts of pollutants have invaded their beloved lake.

Lake Michigan is one of the world's largest lakes, containing by itself some five thousand cubic kilometers of the world's freshwater supply. Thanks to cities like Gary, Indiana, and Chicago, Illinois, the lake has seen heavy industrial pollution, but now those living along its shores are actively fighting for a cleaner lake.

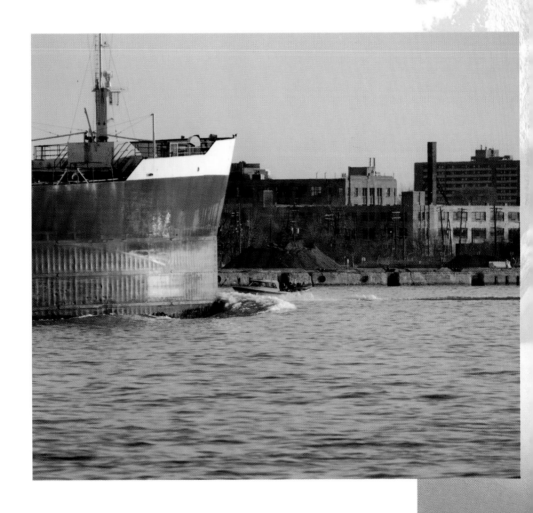

Agriculture

You might begin to think that people in cities are the only ones responsible for water pollution. But that simply isn't true. In fact, pollution from agriculture (mostly found in rural areas) is the leading cause of water source damage. Agricultural activities that cause water pollution include grazing, plowing, pesticide spraying, irrigation, fertilizing, planting, and harvesting. The pollutants that result from these activities include sediment, unwanted nutrients, pathogens, pesticides, and salts. Let's examine how these activities contaminate water sources.

Farmers must constantly monitor runoff from their fields or they risk excessive sedimentation. Erosion and sedimentation occur when wind or water runoff carries soil particles from fields and brings them to a water source. Sedimentation is harmful because it clouds the water,

Irrigation has been around for thousands of years, and as some theorize, was important for the foundations of many civilizations. However, it also encourages and carries agricultural pollution and runoff.

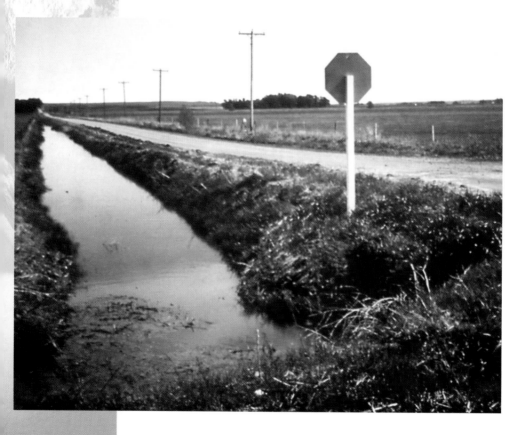

reducing the amount of sunlight able to reach aquatic plants and animals. It also covers fish and clogs their gills, as well as disrupting food supplies.

Erosion also results in unwanted nutrients washing into nearby water sources. Nutrients such as phosphorus, nitrogen, and potassium are all used in fertilizers and applied to crops. When they enter water sources they can cause excessive plant growth, kill fish, and contaminate drinking water.

Confining animals to concentrated plots of land in feed lots is also hazardous to nearby water sources. Runoff from these areas carries bacteria and viruses from the high amounts of feces and other various animal wastes.

Pesticides are chemicals applied to crops to fight off various unwanted organisms: bugs, weeds, or fungi that threaten crops in some way. Unfortunately, many of these pesticides have proved harmful to humans and other life forms. If farmers are not careful in controlling runoff, pesticides can collect and flow towards nearby water sources, where they enter the food chain through fish and plant life that absorb them. After that, they make their way up the food chain and eventually to human beings.

What Pollutants are Found in Runoff?

If you take a moment to think about all the pollutants on an average street in your neighborhood, or in a nearby city, you'll start to realize how many pollutants enter our water from runoff. The following information is from oceansidecleanwaterprogram.org:

- Chemicals like oil, chlorine (used for swimming pools), cleaners, pesticides and fertilizers can harm the animals, bugs and plants that live in the water, and can make people sick when it floats down to the ocean.
- Too many leaves and grass clippings can take the oxygen out of water and suffocate the plants and animals that need oxygen to breathe.

- The waste from our pets is very harmful to our water bodies. Our pets' waste contains dangerous bacteria that can spread diseases to plants, animals and humans that swim in dirty water.
- Soaps and detergents can also take oxygen out of water and suffocate plants and animals. Also, soaps and detergents eat away at the slimy mucus layer that protects fish from diseases and bacteria.

What Is Storm Water Pollution?

Storm water is closely linked to urban runoff. Storm water is what you might guess it is: water generated from heavy rainfall. Urban runoff and storm water are both the product of impervious surfaces. The more pavement and nonporous surfaces we lay down over our world, the more quickly rainfall will enter our surface water sources, bringing with it all the pollutants it has picked up along the way.

In the past, there have been two systems for dealing with storm water: separate and combined sewer systems. Separate systems have two sewer systems—one for storm

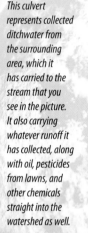

This culvert represents collected ditchwater from the surrounding area, which it has carried to the stream that you see in the picture. It also carrying whatever runoff it has collected, along with oil, pesticides from lawns, and other chemicals straight into the watershed as well.

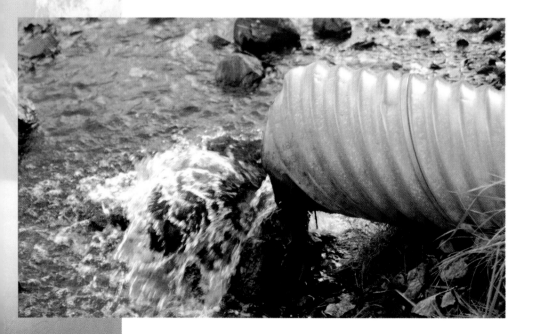

water runoff and another for waste. In these systems, storm water is sent directly to nearby water sources. In combined sewer systems, both waste and storm water are sent to a waste management site—sometimes called a sewage treatment plant—and are then sent back into the water source. However, in this second system, an excess of storm water will overwhelm treatment plants, and then sewage and runoff are both forced back into nearby water sources. Both systems risk contaminating our local water sources with pollutants.

In some cities, deep storage systems are being developed to deal with excess storm water created during heavy rainfall. These deep storage units are massive underground tanks that hold excess storm water until rainfall **subsides**, and then redirect the polluted water towards a waste treatment center. Unfortunately, these systems are extremely expensive to install, and ultimately they deal with the symptoms of storm water without treating its cause— impervious surfaces. Most cities would rather spend large amounts of money on underground reserve tanks than risk halting urban development.

Some cities have shown interest in alternative solutions, however. One such solution is called "green infrastructure." Green infrastructure is basically reintroducing green plants back into urban environments. These cities have begun planting trees and shrubs along their streets and buildings in order to build a network of waterways, wetlands, woodlands, and wildlife habitats. What happens is quite simple: the environment manages storm water naturally, capturing rainfall and absorbing pollutants before they reenter our water sources.

Extreme Situations

In some cases, storm water can quickly become floodwater. Flooding is not a necessarily a problem of developing countries or poor areas with little money. In fact, flooding is more dangerous in developed and urbanized areas where impervious surfaces abound.

Take the city of New Orleans and 2005's hurricane Katrina as an example. Once two or three major **levees** had broken, the city quickly flooded. Some parts of New Orleans were under more than 15 feet of water. Floods cause more damage than storm water to a city's water source, mixing all kinds of sewage, waste, and pollution with fresh water sources. In most extreme cases, the first priority is getting everyone out of the city, but once the waters have receded, cities are faced with the difficult challenge of removing pollutants from their water sources.

What Is Surface Water?

Surface water includes most of what you probably think of as water: all water that is naturally open to the air. This includes lakes, rivers, oceans, reservoirs and any other water sources exposed to the atmosphere—even glaciers.

There are three categories of surface water: permanent (called perennial), semi-permanent (ephemeral) and man-made. Permanent surface waters are sources that are present throughout the year—oceans, most rivers, and swamps. Semi-permanent surface waters only hold water for part of the year—like a seasonal lagoon, or creek. Man-made structures such as dams or reservoirs comprise the third category.

Surface water is replenished (or renewed) naturally by precipitation and lost naturally through **evaporation** and seepage into groundwater. Surface water is where we get the water we need to survive. Water from streams, lakes, and reservoirs is used for a variety of purposes every day.

What is Groundwater?

Groundwater is the water that **saturates** soil and rocks below the surface of the ground. Groundwater, like surface water, is extremely important to the health of the earth and human beings. Consider the following facts about groundwater that are typical of its importance to industry and agriculture in a developed country:

• Scientists estimate groundwater accounts for more than 95% of all fresh water available for use.

• Nearly 95% of rural residents rely on groundwater for their drinking supply.

• About half of irrigated cropland uses groundwater.

• Approximately one third of industrial water needs are fulfilled by using groundwater.

• On average, about 40% of river flow depends on groundwater.

Groundwater exists in a variety of forms beneath the surface of the earth. When a portion of soil or rock holds a quantity of water within it, this is called an **aquifer**. The depth below the surface of the earth at which soil becomes

This field is at full saturation, with water clearly being unable to soak into the ground due to the ground being full already. Another strong rain could cause flooding and subsequent erosion.

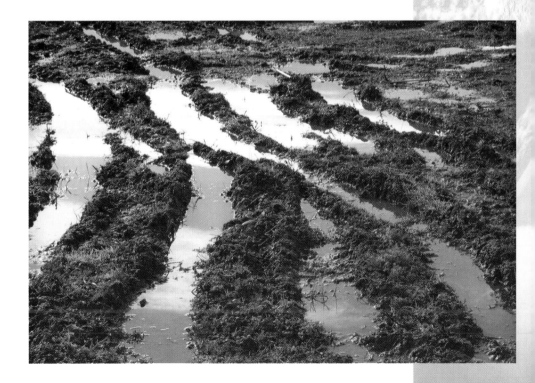

completely saturated with water is called the water table. Groundwater is continually renewed or "recharged" by rivers and lakes.

How Groundwater and Surface Water Interact

Groundwater can feed surface water. An aquifer that is not confined to a rock or sediment is called an unconfined aquifer. An unconfined aquifer that feeds streams is said to provide the stream's base flow. (This is called a gaining stream.)

Similarly, groundwater is fed by precipitation that enters streams and lakes and then filters down below the surface. In some cases, streams actually feed a nearby aquifer—these are called losing streams.

Pollution of Surface and Groundwater Sources

The following four questions and answers outline how we can address pollution in both surface and groundwater sources.

What kind of contamination is it?

Surface water is usually rainwater that collects in surface water bodies, like oceans, lakes, or streams. Another source of surface water is groundwater that discharges to the surface from springs. Surface water pollution occurs when contaminants come into contact and either dissolve or physically mix with the water. Because of the close relationship between sediments and surface water, contaminated sediments are often considered part of surface water contamination. Sediments include the sand and soils on the bottom of an ocean, lake, or stream.

How did it get there?

Surface water can become contaminated in many ways. Surface water can be contaminated when pollutants are discharged directly from an outfall pipe or channel or when they receive contaminated storm water runoff. Direct discharges can come from industrial sources or from certain older sewer systems that overflow during wet weather. Storm water runoff becomes contaminated when rainwater comes into contact with contaminated soil and either dissolves the contamination or carries contaminated soil particles. Surface water can also be contaminated when contaminated groundwater reaches the surface through a spring, or when contaminants in the air are deposited on the surface water. Contaminated soil particles carried by storm water runoff or contaminants from the air can sink to the bottom of a surface water body, mix with the sediment, and remain.

This sewer drain in Minneapolis, Minnesota is a perfect example of surface water pollution. The sewer is contaminated by sewage, and the outflow has caused a large algae bloom upon the water of the Mississippi River.

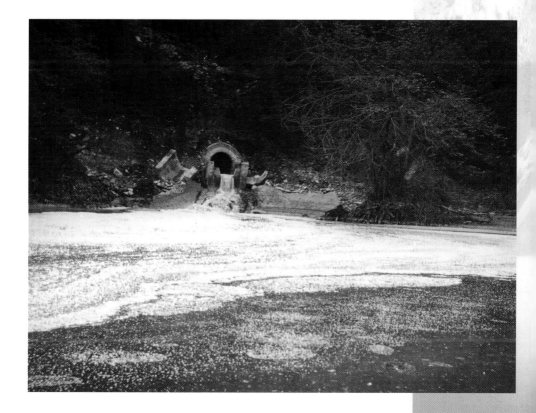

How does it hurt animals, plants and humans?

A change in the water chemistry due to surface water contamination can negatively affect all levels of an ecosystem. It can impact the health of lower food chain organisms and, consequently, the availability of the food supply up through the food chain. It can also impact the health of wetlands and impair their ability to support healthy ecosystems, control flooding, and filter pollutants from storm water runoff. Contaminated surface water can also affect the health of animals and humans when they drink or bathe in contaminated water or, for aquatic organisms, when they ingest contaminated sediments. One of the major concerns associated with contaminated surface water is the ability of aquatic organisms, like fish, to accumulate and concentrate contaminants in their bodies. When other animals or humans ingest these organisms,

This well has flooded with water that is rich in contaminants from a farmer's field. Due to the poor construction of the well, the floodwaters contaminated the wellhead and leached into the groundwater below.

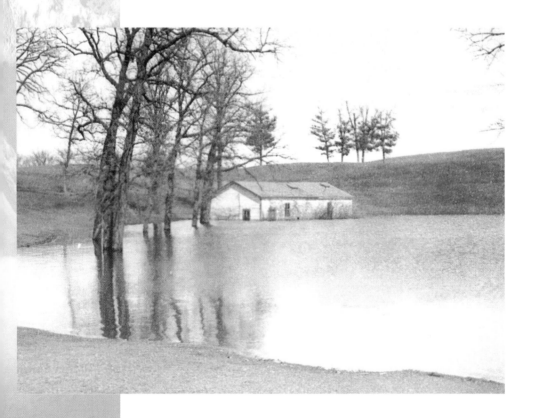

they receive a much higher dose of contamination than they would have if they had been directly exposed to the original source of the contamination.

How can we clean it up?

The most effective approach for cleaning up contaminated surface water is to prevent further discharges from contaminated sources and enable natural biological, chemical, and physical processes to break down the existing contamination. In some surface water bodies where natural processes are not enough to break down the contaminants, other cleanup approaches such as mixing and aeration may be required to further promote natural cleanup. A significant source of surface water contamination may be contaminated sediments. Contaminated sediments generally contain **persistent** contaminants and are difficult to clean up. Three main approaches to cleaning up contaminated sediments are: 1) remove them by dredging; 2) place a cover over them to prevent contact with the surface water; or 3) allow natural processes to cover them or break them down over time. For contamination that does not mix with surface water and floats on the surface, such as that encountered during an oil spill, contamination can be removed by skimming it from the surface using a "boom."

STRAIGHT FROM THE SOURCE

From the United States Environmental Protection Agency document, Economic Benefits Of Runoff Controls

Urbanization also leads to loss of pervious areas (porous surfaces) that allow rainwater to soak into the ground. This can increase the amount and velocity of rainwater flowing to streams and rivers. This increased speed and volume of water can have many impacts, including eroded stream banks, increased turbidity and pollution, increased stream water temperature, and increased water flow. All of these can have an adverse effect on the fish and other organisms living in the stream and the receiving waters. When rainwater cannot soak into the ground, the result can be a loss of drinking water because many areas of the country rely on rainwater soaking into the ground to replenish underground drinking water supplies. Loss of trees due to urbanization can have negative impacts.

Trees are important for controlling the water temperature along the shorelines of water bodies. Since many aquatic plant and animal species are sensitive to changes in water temperature (trout, for example), it is important to keep stream temperatures as close to natural levels as possible. When the shade of trees is lost, the water temperature can increase. "Best management practices," or BMPs, help address these impacts. BMPs are designed to help reduce the amount of pollution in urban runoff. Some help to control the volume and speed of runoff before it enters receiving waters. Many help to increase the amount of rainwater that soaks into the ground to restore groundwater. There are two general types of BMPs: structural and non structural. Structural controls involve building at "facility" for controlling urban runoff. There are a variety of structural controls and most require some level of routine maintenance.

This report discusses two types of structural controls that have been documented as providing economic benefits: urban runoff ponds and constructed wetlands. Non structural BMPs do not require construction of a facility. For example, planning a development so that there are buffers along stream banks and minimizing the amount of impervious area are types of non structural controls. Structural and non structural controls can be used in combination to manage runoff. Urban runoff management controls are now widely accepted due to lessons learned from not planning properly for the impacts associated with increased urbanization. Most local governments require some form of urban runoff management for new development. They require such controls for two reasons: to prevent pollution and to prevent flooding caused by increased runoff, mostly from impervious areas. Usually they require structural controls although some local governments give credit for non structural controls.

What Do You Think?

- Why is it important to design urban runoff treatment management for new developments?

- What are the two types of management practices?

- What are the possible long-term effects of a simple loss of trees beside a stream?

Find Out More

Effects of Pollution on Runoff
www.epa.gov/weatherchannel/stormwater.html#effects

Run Off
ga.water.usgs.gov/edu/watercyclerunoff.html

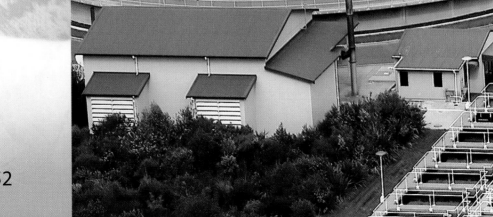

Here's what you need to know

- Untreated wastewater can seriously harm the environment and impact human health.
- The challenge of wastewater management is increasing due to the age of many facilities, population growth, and new environmental contaminants.
- There are various physical, biological, and chemical processes used in wastewater treatment.
- Millions of people around the world, especially children, face serious health risks due to untreated wastewater.

Words to Understand

Effluent is water that flows from a sewage treatment plant after it has been treated.

Grey water is wastewater from clothes washing machines, showers, bathtubs, hand washing, lavatories and sinks.

A **cesspool** is a covered hole or pit for receiving drainage or sewage.

Menstruation is the monthly flow of blood from the uterus of women, beginning at puberty in girls.

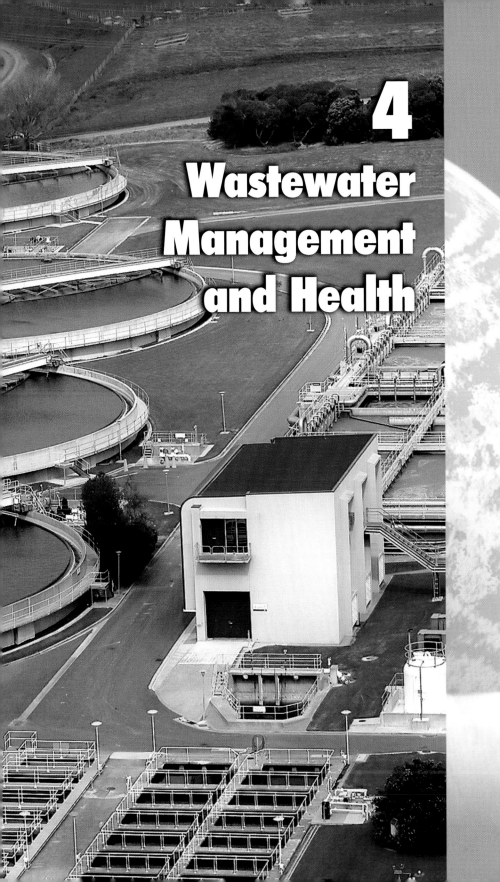

4

Wastewater Management and Health

What is Wastewater?

Wastewater is water that has been used by homes, communities, farms, and businesses that contains enough harmful material to damage the water's quality. Included in wastewater are both domestic sewage and industrial waste from manufacturing sources. Metals, organic pollutants, sediment, bacteria and viruses may all be found in wastewater. As you can probably imagine, untreated wastewater can seriously harm the environment and human beings.

Why is Wastewater Management Necessary?

Wastewater treatment is needed so that we can safely use our water sources. Everything from fishing and swimming to drinking and bathing require waters that are clean and safe. You might be surprised to learn that as recent as the early 20th century, much of the world's waters (especially urban waters) were contaminated. In those days, the primary concern of waste management was keeping human waste out of water sources. Most people in the world then (and many still today) had little or no means of disposing

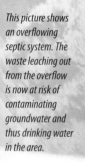

This picture shows an overflowing septic system. The waste leaching out from the overflow is now at risk of contaminating groundwater and thus drinking water in the area.

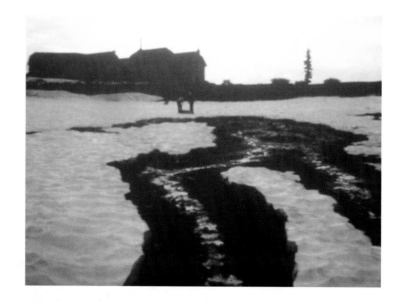

of waste safely. They most often used some form of the **cesspool** for their wastewater.

As the population in most countries grew, so did the amount of wastewater produced—especially in highly populated cities. People could no longer safely dispose of wastewater in cesspools and local water sources. Diseases from improper waste disposal were killing many people in the cities of the world. It was clear that a new system would be needed for managing waste.

What are the Challenges of Waste Management?

The EPA lists the following as current challenges to wastewater management:

• Many of the wastewater treatment and collection facilities are now old and worn, and require further improvement, repair or replacement to maintain their useful life;

• The character and quantity of contaminants presenting problems today are far more complex than those that presented challenges in the past;

• Population growth is taxing many existing wastewater treatment systems and creating a need for new plants;

• Farm runoff and increasing urbanization provide additional sources of pollution not controlled by wastewater treatment; and

• One third of new development is served by decentralized systems (e.g., septic systems) as population migrates further from metropolitan areas.

Of course, pollutants are the primary challenge of wastewater management. Pollutants can perhaps be best understood in five categories: oxygen-demanding substances, pathogens, nutrients, synthetic-organic/inorganic chemicals, and thermal threats.

The first category, oxygen-demanding substances, may require some background information. You see, dissolved oxygen is a key element of water and is necessary to support aquatic life. Many substances in **effluent** quickly use up oxygen. These substances include organic matter and chemicals from domestic sewage and agricultural and industrial waste. Usually these oxygen-demanding substances are destroyed or converted to other compounds by bacteria—if there is sufficient oxygen in the water. But in the process of breaking down these substances, a significant portion of the dissolved oxygen is lost, leaving little for aquatic life.

Pathogens also pose a threat to wastewater management. Pathogens are infectious microorganisms that carry diseases such as typhoid fever, cholera, and dysentery—all of which are a major threat in parts of the world without proper waste treatment facilities. Pathogens are carried into surface and groundwater by sewage from cities and industrial wastes, as well as storm runoff. Fortunately, most waste management facilities have means of killing these organisms—chlorination of water being the most

Taken to showcase the poor conditions in a Depression era migrant workers camp, this photo shows what happens with poor sanitation conditions. This septic system has failed completely, releasing its collection of laundry, latrine, and shower water and permitting the growth of all sorts of bacteria and other pathogens that may now affect the quality of the workers' water.

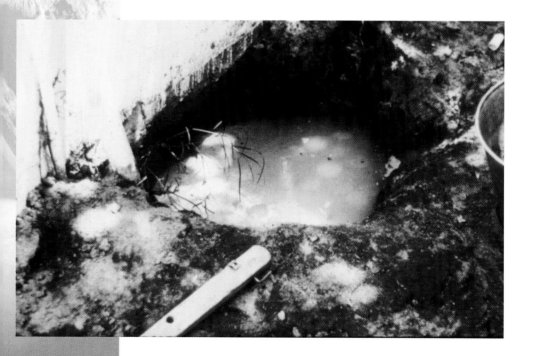

popular.

Many nutrients found in water are essential to living organisms, but when these same nutrients appear in too large a quantity, they can become harmful to our environment and health. Large amounts of these nutrients are the result of sewage, certain industrial wastes, and drainage from fertilized land. These nutrients overstimulate the growth of water plants and algae, which can interfere with normal aquatic life. Too much algae or water plants can block out sunlight and take away oxygen that other plants and animals need to survive. They can also cause unpleasant tastes and odors in drinking water.

Inorganic and synthetic organic chemicals include a wide range of chemicals that can threaten our health and environment. Included in this category are detergents, household cleaning aids, heavy metals, pharmaceuticals, synthetic organic pesticides and herbicides, industrial chemicals, and the wastes from their manufacture. These substances can be toxic to fish and aquatic life and many are harmful to humans—even in very small quantities.

Thermal threats in wastewater are the result of heat, which can reduce the capacity of water to retain oxygen. Unfortunately, even if water has been properly treated and cleaned in a waste management facility, it can still pose a threat to our environment and health if its temperature is higher than the receiving body of water's temperature. Water from sewage systems and treatment plants will often elevate the temperature of the receiving body of water, which can harm the surrounding ecosystem.

How is Waste Management Done?

The most common form of pollution control in the United States consists of a system of sewers and wastewater treatment plants. The sewers collect municipal wastewater from homes, businesses, and industries and deliver it to facilities for treatment before it is discharged to water bodies or land, or reused. Most often, these are centralized plants that collect all the wastewater for an entire region or city.

Many of the earliest sewer systems were combined sewers, which collect both sanitary wastewater and storm water runoff in a single system. These systems brought all wastewater to a centralized waste management site, and were thought to be the best way to manage wastewater. We know now, however, that the overflow system built into combined sewer systems can be dangerous. If rainfall pushes the level of water in these sewer systems too high, they have special overflows designed to release excess flow into nearby water sources. This means that all the pathogens and pollutants are also released into the water source.

Because of the combined sewer system's flaws, many cities have developed sanitary sewers, designed to carry wastewater from domestic, industrial and commercial sources, but not to carry storm water. These systems carry wastewater to a waste management facility, where the following three basic processes are applied: physical, biological, and chemical.

Physical Processes

Physical processes were some of the earliest to be used by waste management specialists. Their action is still fairly simple today, although the technology used has become increasingly sophisticated. The basic function of these physical processes is to remove solids from wastewater. They do so using screens, which remove debris and solids, but they also use gravity to allow heavier solids to settle and remove them that way. Some particles with entrapped air will float to the top of the water and can also be removed. Today, incredibly advanced screens with micro-sized pores block even the smallest bits of matter from passing through.

Biological Processes

Very much a pleasant surprise, it seems that some bacteria can actually be cultivated to consume organic matter in sewage, turning it into new bacterial cells, carbon dioxide, and other, safer by-products. In the 1920s, scientists discovered that we could accelerate this "natural" cleaning process by adding massive amounts of oxygen to waste management systems in order to remove organic material from wastewater. With the addition of oxygen, large numbers of microorganisms (bacteria) grew and rapidly devoured organic pollutants. The left over bacteria was removed by physical processes, leaving much cleaner water when all was done.

Chemical Processes

Some chemicals can be added to wastewater to create changes in pollutants that allow physical processes to more easily remove them. Chemicals such as alum, lime, or iron salts can be added to wastewater to cause certain pollutants—such as phosphorus—to bunch together into

Raw sewage pours untreated from a factory's outlet into the Mississippi River. Note how the milky white color of the water is evident even in this black and white photo.

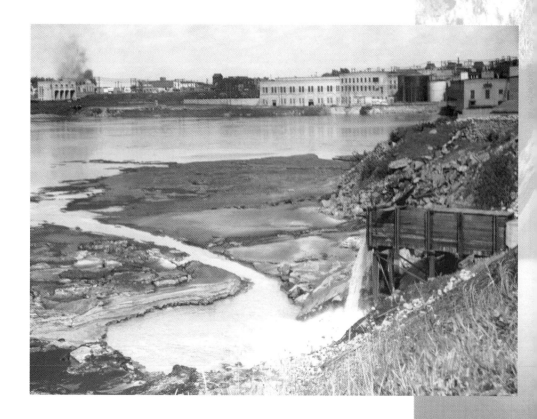

larger, heavier masses that are blocked by physical screens. The waste management industry has recently developed certain synthetic inert chemicals known as polymers that are able to further bunch pollutants together. Synthetic inert chemicals are chemicals that do not react readily with other chemicals, meaning they are largely safe for human beings and the environment.

Sanitation

When you hear people talking about waste management issues, you will very likely also hear them talking about sanitation. Sanitation is an issue closely tied to wastewater management. Sanitation is the word used to describe the ways in which we try to protect public health from waste. Wherever humans gather, their waste will accumulate, and probably their water source will be affected. The more progress we make toward better sanitation, the better our health and environment. Not just human beings are affected by wastewater, after all, but so is every other species that comes into contact with it.

Wastewater can harm us in the following ways:

- By polluting drinking water
- By entering the food chain through fish and shellfish, fruits, vegetables, and other plant life
- By contaminating water for activities like bathing and swimming
- By creating breeding sites for flies, insects, and bacteria that can spread disease

Sanitation is a very big issue facing the world today. In 2004, only 59 percent of the world population had access to any type of improved sanitation facility. Put another way, 4 out of 10 people in the world have no access to improved sanitation. Improved sanitation can be as simple as a working toilet or a sink with clean water. Investing in improved sanitation could save millions of lives, as well as millions of dollars. But often sanitation is overlooked for more short-term profit-earning enterprises.

Who is at Risk?

Almost everyone in the developing world is still at risk of poor sanitation. But it turns out that children and women are particularly at risk among all populations. Studies have shown that the provision of safe water and sanitation facilities is a necessary first step for proper learning environments to be established. Sanitation provides women, who are often the primary caregivers to children, greater privacy and support for maintaining children's health. And schools that have sanitation facilities are able to attract and keep more students—especially girls. Studies show that **menstruating** girls are reluctant to attend schools without toilets, and their parents are less likely to force them to attend. Of course, there is the added benefit that children with proper sanitation are much more healthy and therefore much more able to learn and further the development of themselves and their community. Consider these facts and figures from UNICEF:

- One in four girls does not complete primary school, compared with one in seven boys.
- Girls bear the burden of water collection, which can take many hours a day, leaving them with no time or energy for school.
- A study by the government of Bangladesh and UNICEF revealed an 11% increase in girls' enrollment mainly due to the provision of sanitary facilities.

STRAIGHT FROM THE SOURCE

From the Unicef document, Sanitation is Vital for Health

Human feces are the primary source of diarrheal pathogens. Without sanitation facilities to safely contain and dispose of human feces, the health of everyone living nearby is put at risk. Diarrheal disease is a leading cause of under five child mortality and can be reduced by improved sanitation. Additionally, worm infections impair children's health, nutrition and cognitive development. Children weakened by diarrhea are more susceptible to other infections, namely respiratory infections, which are another leading cause of child mortality. Sanitation affects children's development and futures.

Supporting facts and figures:

- Daily child deaths under age five from diarrheal diseases in 2004: 5000 (Progress for Children (PFC) 6, UNICEF 2006).

- % of diarrheal deaths related to lack of water and sanitation: 88% (PFC 6).

- % of total under five child mortality due to diarrhea : 17%, not including neonatal diarrhea (WHO 2005, CHERG).

- Diarrheal-related deaths per year of children under 5: 1.5 million (PFC 6).

- Children under 18 without access to improved sanitation: 980 million, 280 million of which are children under five. (UNICEF, 2006).

- Ratio by which improved sanitation and hygiene reduces diarrhea-related deaths: 2/3 (PFC 5).

- Diarrhea as proportionate cause of child mortality: 2nd highest single cause after pneumonia (WHO 2005, CHERG).

What Do You Think?

- Why is sanitation so important?

- Why do you think worm infections affect cognitive development?

- What does sanitation include, do you think?

Find Out More

International Year of Sanitation
esa.un.org/iys

Water-Related Disease
www.who.int/water_sanitation_health/diseases/en/index.html

World Water Day
www.unwater.org/worldwaterday/flashindex.html

Here's what you need to know

- Seventeen percent of the world's population does not have access to safe drinking water.
- Adequate access to drinking water is defined as 20 liters of safe water from an "improved" source per person per day within 1 kilometer of the person's home.
- Contaminated water is the largest cause of sickness and death worldwide.
- Microorganisms in drinking water form the greatest threat to public health.
- There are few chemical contaminants that pose a risk in single exposures.
- Infants, children and pregnant women are most at risk from chemical contaminants in drinking water.
- Bottled water is not necessarily safer—in some cases it is actually more dangerous.

Words to Understand

A public **standpipe** is a vertical pipe extending up from a water supply.

A **borehole** is a shaft drilled deep into the ground so that safe water may be drawn from below the surface.

DALYs are Disability-Adjusted Life Years that consider disease burden due to death and disability in a single measurement, rather than separately.

Renal refers to anything relating to the kidneys.

Anemia is an illness in which the blood does not have enough red blood cells.

Electrolytes are charged atoms that regulate metabolic processes, such as the flow of nutrients into and waste products out of cells.

The inside of the small intestines are lined with **villi**, which are slender, finger-shaped processes that help absorb nutrients.

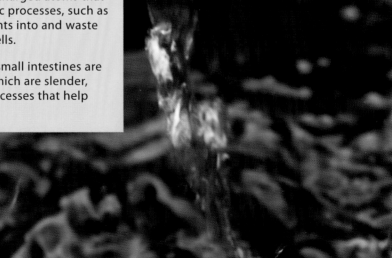

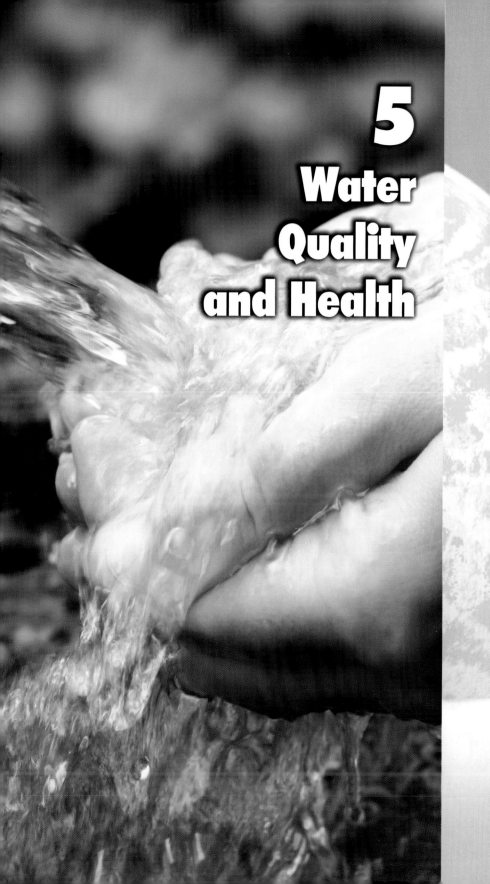

5
Water Quality and Health

Everyone needs water to survive. Water is an essential part of our daily diets. Unfortunately, as of 2004 an average of 17 percent of the world's population does not have access to "improved" water sources. When only rural populations are considered, 27 percent of the world's rural population is without access to adequate safe water supply.

Definition of Access for Safe Water Supply

The Joint Monitoring Programme (JMP) of the World Health Organization and the United Nations, defines access to safe water as the availability of at least 20 liters (5.28 gal) per person per day from an "improved" source within 1 kilometer (.62 mi) of a user's home. An "improved" source of water is one that is likely to provide safe, contaminant-free drinking water.

Improved Sources

- household connection
- public **standpipe**
- **borehole**

This slide shows a slum in Ecuador that was heavily affected by cholera due to its proximity to unsafe water sources.

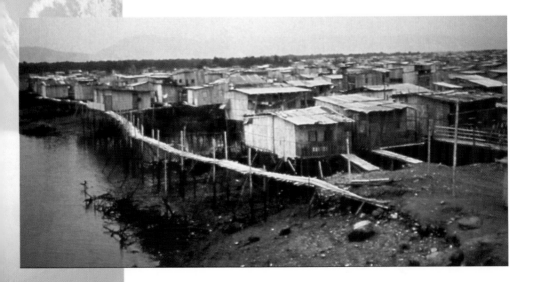

- protected dug well
- protected spring
- rainwater collection

Not improved Sources

- unprotected well
- unprotected spring
- vendor provided water
- bottled water
- tanker truck water

Where does drinking water come from?

Depending on where you are in the world, your drinking water comes from different sources. In the developed world countries most people in both urban and rural areas can turn on a tap in the kitchen for a glass of fresh cold water. According to the Joint Monitoring Programme (JMP) of the WHO and UNICEF, as of 2004, 99 percent of the population in the developed world countries had access to safe water supply. Of these, 99 percent of the population in urban areas and 89 percent of the population in rural areas had an in-house connect.

In developing world countries 80 percent of the population had access to adequate clean water in 2004, according to the JMP. In urban areas, 70 percent of the population had an in-house connect, but in rural areas, only 25 percent of the population obtained water through in-house connects.

Where does tap water come from?

In-house connections carry water into houses from many different sources depending on where in the world you live. In urban areas water is usually drawn from surface water sources, such as lakes, rivers, and reservoirs. In

Ask the Doctor

Q: When I get a glass of water from the tap at my brother's apartment, the water looks all white and cloudy at first. It eventually clears up, but it makes me nervous-is it safe to drink?

Without knowing more information, I can't say for sure whether the water at your brother's apartment is free from any toxins. I can tell you, however, that the white cloudy appearance is due to lots of tiny bubbles that come out when the water is first expelled from the faucet.

rural areas, people are more likely to drink ground water pumped from a well. The wells tap into underground aquifers—the natural fresh water storage areas under the earth's surface—that may range in size from a few square kilometers to thousands of square kilometers.

Poor water quality is a serious public health concern. According to the 2006 UN Global Environment Outlook Report, contaminated water is the largest cause of sickness and death worldwide. There are many different contaminants found in water supplies around the world. The following is only a small sample of common contaminants found in drinking water and their various health effects:

Microorganisms

Microorganisms in drinking water pose a major worldwide health threat. In fact, infectious diseases caused by bacteria, viruses, protozoa and parasitic worms (*helminths*) are the most common health risk associated with drinking water. According to WHO, diarrheal disease amounts to an estimated 4.1 percent of the total **DALY** global burden of disease and is responsible for the deaths of 1.8 million people every year. Gastrointestinal illnesses are the most common routes of infection for all the waterborne pathogens, though a few travel via water droplets in the air (*Legionella*), and a couple of others enter the body through mucous membranes or broken skin during bathing (*Schistosoma).*

BACTERIA

Escherichia coli pathogenic strains (E.coli)

E. coli are part of the normal bacteria flora present in the intestines of humans and animals; they are normally harmless. However, when ingested in drinking water, *E. coli* can cause mild to severe gastrointestinal illness. Children under 5 years of age are at risk for developing haemolytic uraemic syndrome (HUS), which is characterized by acute **renal** failure and **anemia**. *E. coli* are known as indicator organisms because their presence indicates the presence of fecal matter and therefore other dangerous bacteria in the water. Water intended for use as drinking water should contain no indicator organisms.

Salmonella typhi

Salmonella bacteria can be divided into two categories—typhoidal and nontyphoidal. *Salmonella typhi* is a typhoidal species that has a gastrointestinal route of infection. There are four possible disease presentations: 1) a carrier state with no symptoms, 2) mild to severe gastrointestinal illness 3) high fever with positive blood tests and 4) typhoid fever (long-lasting fever, with/without diarrhea). Typhoid fever is still a serious concern in areas without adequate sanitation. *E.coli* can be used as indictors of *Salmonella* presence or absence.

Vibrio cholerae

Vibrio cholerae, cholera, has a gastrointestinal route of infection and causes severe loose and watery diarrhea. The diarrhea is so severe that the infection may cause a patient to lose as much as 10–15 liters (2.64-3.96 gal) of liquid

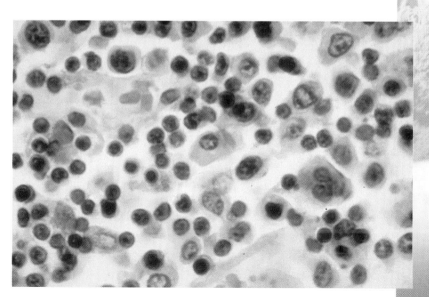

Although vaccine for typhoid fever has been in existence since the late nineteenth century, outbreaks still occur around the world. One recent outbreak in the Congo killed hundreds of people.

per day. As a result of the loss of fluid, as many as 60% of untreated patients die as a result of severe dehydration and loss of **electrolytes**. *V. cholerae* outbreaks are usually the result of poor sanitation, but they have been found in water with no *E. coli*, so *E. coli* cannot be used as indicators of their presence.

VIRUSES
Hepatitis A

Hepatitis A (HAV) enters the body via the gastrointestinal tract and then gets into the bloodstream where it travels to the liver and can cause severe damage to liver cells. The virus is more dangerous to people over 50 years of age. HAV enters drinking water supply through a combination of fecal matter from infected individuals and poor sanitation.

Rotaviruses

Rotaviruses are the largest cause of infant death in the world. The viruses infect the **villi** of the small intestines and cause severe watery diarrhea, fever, abdominal pain and vomiting. If untreated, the resulting dehydration and loss of electrolytes can lead to death. Drinking water is not the most common route of transmission, but it is still a risk. *E. coli* are not a reliable indicator of their presence.

PROTOZOA
Entamoeba histoltyica

Entamoeba histolytica is the most common intestinal protozoan pathogen worldwide. Symptoms of amoebic dysentery include diarrhea (often bloody, or with mucus), cramping, and fever. The protozoa can also enter other organs, such as the liver, lungs or brain, which can prove deadly. Contaminated drinking water is a confirmed source for *E. histolytica* and *E. coli* is not a reliable indicator of its presence.

HELMINTHS

Dracunculus medinensis

D. medinensis, more commonly called guinea worm, is the only nematode transmitted through drinking water. Larvae are swallowed in drinking water and then grow within the body (females up to 700 mm (27.56 in). When the female reaches full size, she puts her head out through a blister or cut on the infected person's foot or leg when he is standing in the water and releases her larvae to begin the cycle anew. Symptoms occur just before this stage and include hives, redness of the skin, shortness of breath, vomiting, giddiness, and itchiness. In some cases, the opening where the worm is exiting the body becomes infected. The worm is limited to an area of sub-Saharan Africa, and is spread though contaminated drinking water supplies.

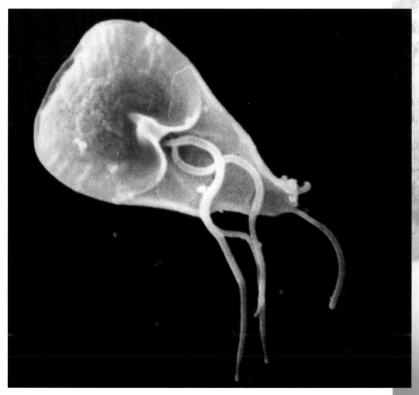

This is a protozoa of the genus Giardia, which is a water-borne parasite often referred to as "beaver fever," as that particular mammal is one of its most common vectors. Giardia is infamous for giving its victims vomiting and diarrhea at the same time.

Treatment of water for microorganisms

Drinking water is treated for microorganisms mainly through the use of various filtering systems or through chemical disinfection with chlorine, monochloramine, or chlorine dioxide. Each process has varying success rates with each specific type of pathogen. The single most important step in removing the risk of microbial contamination from water supply is increasing worldwide access to adequate sanitation. For these reasons, UNICEF promotes sanitation and simple hygiene, like hand washing as the first line of defense for protecting drinking water from contamination.

Chemicals

Unlike microbial organisms, there are few chemicals in drinking water that can lead to health problems after only a single exposure. Instead, health problems that result from exposure to chemically contaminated drinking water

Entamoeba is one of the most common amoeboid infections encountered in the world. Although most of the time it only affects the gastrointestinal tract, it can migrate to the nerves and brain, where it literally consumes them.

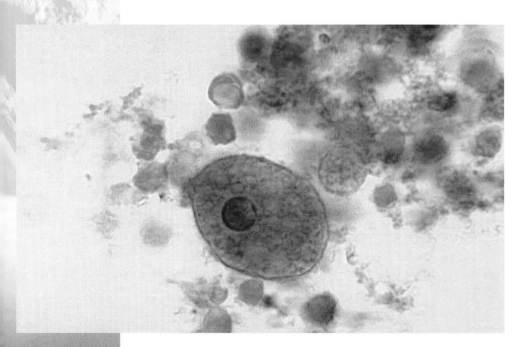

are the result or long-term exposure, or bioaccumulation of the chemicals within the body. Infants, young children and pregnant women are most at risk from these chemical contaminants.

Arsenic

Arsenic is a naturally occurring contaminant that is present at safe levels in most areas of the world. It is present in higher amounts in certain areas of the world, such as India and Bangladesh. It is introduced into drinking-water sources primarily through the dissolution of naturally occurring minerals and ores. Even though it is not a human-made pollutant, its presence in drinking water sources can still cause serious health problems. Long-term exposure, even to low concentrations, can cause painful skin lesions and can result in cancers of the skin, lungs, bladder and kidney. Concentrations in drinking water can be controlled because they are usually dependent on how deep a well is dug.

Fluoride

Like, arsenic, fluoride is a naturally occurring contaminant that is a concern in India and Bangladesh. The effects of fluoride are usually only visible after prolonged exposure. Fluorosis will lead to severe crippling and ultimately death.

Lead

Lead is not a "raw" drinking water issue, but a problem found in houses with in-house connections. Lead is sometimes present in household plumbing systems containing lead in pipes, solder, fittings, or the service connections to homes. The amount of lead in the water depends on the pH, temperature, water hardness, and standing time of the water, with soft, acidic water yielding the highest lead concentrations. Infants, children, and pregnant women are at the highest risk of absorption and accumulation of lead in the skeleton. Lead accumulation can eventually lead to neurological and behavioral effects.

Other Trace Metals

Trace metals such as mercury, copper, selenium, and zinc are essential to humans in low concentrations. However, exposure to high levels, or prolonged exposure, which can lead to bioaccumulation, can be a health hazard. Mining and industry can increase concentrations above what would occur naturally in drinking water.

Sediment

Sediment in drinking water is not necessarily harmful itself, but it may be harboring other contaminants. In countries where sediment is an issue, people allow water to sit, so that the sediment can settle to the bottom of water vessels before the water is consumed.

Other Chemical Contaminants

Pesticides

Organic chemicals and pesticides like DDT travel into drinking water with agricultural run off. Nitrate and nitrite, both arising from excessive application of fertilizers, have been associated with anemia in bottle-fed infants.

Is Bottled Water Better Water?

In many areas of the world, people are reaching for a bottle of water believing it to be a safer option than water from their faucet. But is this really true? The World Health Organization argues that certain factors can be more easily controlled in the packaging process and therefore bottles of water might be a safer option. For example, concentrations of lead may be more easily controlled in bottles than in piped systems of water. However, bottled water is not sterile water, and other factors, such as microorganisms may be harder to control than in piped systems. In addition, there have been cases of fraud of which consumers need to be aware. In summary, there is no short answer to the question of whether the water itself is safer, but the plastic bottles generate a large amount of waste.

Real People

Source: www.peacecorps.gov/wws/educators/enrichment/africa/countries/mauritania/source1.html

Heather Cameron is a volunteer with the Peace Corps in Rosso, Mauritania. The Senegal River serves as water source for Heather and the 50,000 people living in Rosso.

A government utility company pipes water from the river into an underground system through the town. Each neighborhood has several corner faucets where young women and children can fill up their buckets for a few pennies. More fortunate families have a faucet, or even a shower, in their homes.

The water contains a lot of sediment from the river, but people let it sit overnight so that the sediment settles to the bottom. Heather also says it is important to filter and treat the water (which the utility company says it does) to guard against illnesses like giarda and to kill amoebas.

Iron

Iron does not cause any serious health problems, but in high concentrations it tastes very unpleasant. As a result, if safe water is rich in iron, many people turn back to older, unsafe, but better-tasting water sources.

How much is safe?

The World Health Organization has developed guideline values for many chemicals found in drinking water. A guideline value represents the concentration of a chemical that does not result in any significant risk to health over a lifetime of consumption.

STRAIGHT FROM THE SOURCE

From the UNICEF document, Arsenic Mitigation in Bangladesh

Nearly 40,000 people showing the skin lesions symptoms characteristic of arsenicosis have been identified in Bangladesh. While there is a long latency of more than 20 years, lesions can appear more quickly if arsenic concentrations are very high. However, these symptoms are usually reversible if detected early and people stop drinking arsenic-contaminated water. Long-term exposure to arsenic can cause serious health problems including internal cancers of the skin, lungs, bladder and kidney, which can be fatal. These cancers can occur without the skin lesions. Most of the deaths caused by arsenic are expected to be from lung cancer. Studies have shown exposure to arsenic contaminated water can also cause impaired cognitive development in children.

Social Impacts

People with arsenic poisoning suffer enormous social stigma in Bangladesh. Many people believe arsenic poisoning is contagious or a curse. Parents are reluctant to let their children play with children suffering arsenic poisoning and patients can be shunned within their villages. For women, the situation is worse. In Bangladesh, a woman's attractiveness lies in her beauty, which is often judged by her pale complexion. This makes it harder, in some cases impossible, for single women suffering from arsenic poisoning to marry. Once married, women face the risk of divorce if they develop arsenicosis skin lesions. This can be a dire situation in Bangladesh's male dominated society, where unmarried women are more vulnerable to poverty and social exclusion. Women are also less likely to receive early diagnosis or treatment.

Limited options

In some arsenic-affected areas there are relatively few safe water options available. Some alternatives are safer, but less convenient, than arsenic-contaminated shallow tube wells. It is hard to compete with the low-cost, easy maintenance and convenience of shallow tube wells.

Changing Behavior

Previous actions to encourage people to switch from surface water to groundwater in order to reduce diarrheal disease were phenomenally effective: some 97 per cent of the rural population relies on tube wells for drinking water. This success has now created a new challenge, as people are not interested in switching from tube wells to other arsenic-free sources. Even though the arsenic contamination in river or pond water is negligible, if untreated it could still contain diarrhea-carrying bacteria. Arsenic has no taste, odor or color, and poses only long-term health risks, unlike the immediate risks of diarrhea.

What Do You Think?

• What are the obstacles to getting people to switch water sources?

• What do you think will be the most effective way to reeducate the people of Bangladesh about healthy water sources?

• What are the social stigmas of arsenic poisoning for women? Are these social values unique to Bangladesh?

Find Out More

Ceramic Filters in Myanmar
www.unicef.org/infobycountry/myanmar_40738.html

UNICEF
www.unicef.org/wes/index_43106.html

World Health Organization
www.who.int/water_sanitation_health/dwq/en/

Here's what you need to know

- The world needs to work together to protect water resources and ensure safe water access for all.
- In 2000 the UN Millennium Development Goals were agreed upon, to end poverty, hunger, disease, illiteracy, environmental destruction, and discrimination against women by 2015.
- In 2002, at the World Summit on Sustainable Development, world leaders agreed to end destruction of aquatic diversity.
- The UN declared 2005-2015 the Decade for Action: "Water for Life."
- The UN declared 2008 the International Year of Sanitation.
- The 2008 World Water Week focused on the global sanitation crisis.
- As part of emergency water response, UNICEF provides clean water through small water purification systems donated by the Norwegian government.
- You can join in the efforts to solve issues of water pollution, sanitation, water quality and health by getting involved with organizations, or by taking some simple personal steps.

Words to Understand

A person's **posterity** is their children and descendents.

When an action is **unprecedented**, nothing like it has ever been done before.

The **exploitation** of resources is to make use of resources unfairly, to the advantage of only one group.

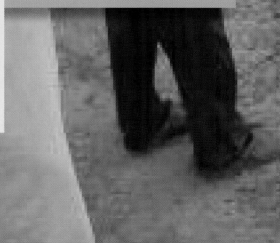

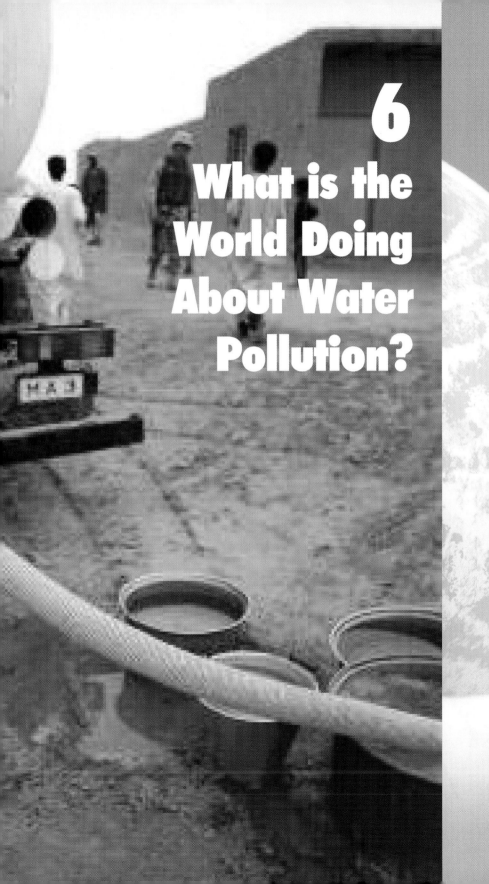

6

What is the World Doing About Water Pollution?

Since water is one of the world's most valuable and vital resources, it stands to reason that the world should stand together to fight against issues of water pollution, water scarcity, sanitation and public health, and loss of coastal ecosystems and aquatic biodiversity. Sometimes the major issues of human water requirements and preserving the natural environment seem to conflict, but in the end all goals aim toward more sustainable use of improved water sources that will be better for both our **posterity** and the planet.

Millennium Development Goals

At the United Nations Millennium Summit in September 2000 leaders from around the world met and agreed to set goals for fighting and ending world poverty, hunger, disease, illiteracy, environmental destruction, and discrimination against women by the year 2015. This discussion became the Millennium Development Goals (MDGs), eight goals around which all United Nations programs now operate. The MDGs have now been agreed to by all countries in the world and act as a framework that forms the base of **unprecedented** efforts to meet the needs of all the people on Earth. The Millennium Development Goals are:

1. Eradicate extreme hunger and poverty
2. Achieve universal primary education
3. Promote gender equality and empower women
4. Reduce child mortality
5. Improve maternal health
6. Combat HIV/AIDS, malaria, and other diseases
7. Ensure environmental sustainability
8. Develop a global partnership for development.

Water quality management is related to achieving all eight goals, but it is most closely tied to the objectives of Goal 7:

- countries should encourage new sustainable development and halt the loss of environmental resources as a result of existing development;
- halve by 2015 the proportion of people without sustainable access to safe drinking water and basic sanitation;
- reduce biodiversity loss by 2010; and
- achieve improvements in the lives of at least 100 million slum dwellers by 2020.

2002 World Summit on Sustainable Development

At this summit in Johannesburg, South Africa, in addition to the MDG of halving the proportion of people lacking access to safe drinking water and basic sanitation by 2015, countries committed themselves to achieving a significant reduction in the rate of biodiversity loss in aquatic ecosystems by 2010.

Water for life

In December 2003 the United Nations General Assembly declared the years 2005 to 2015 as the International Decade for Action: "Water for Life."

The primary goal of the "Water for Life" Decade is to fulfill the Millennium Development Goals of halving the proportion of people without access to safe drinking water and basic sanitation by 2015, and to stop unsustainable use and exploitation of water resources.

Some of the important issues on which the Water for Life decade will focus include:

- water scarcity
- access to sanitation and health
- water and gender

Did You Know?

A total of about 20 million square kilometers of land and sea have been placed under protection worldwide as of 2006. This is an area more than twice the size of China. However, only about 2 million square kilometers are marine ecosystems, despite their important role in the sustainability of fish stocks and of coastal livelihoods.

- environment and biodiversity
- disaster prevention
- food and agriculture
- pollution and energy

As women play important roles in getting and managing water resources, a special emphasis will be placed on the involvement of women in these efforts.

International Year of Sanitation

The United Nations declared 2008 as the International Year of Sanitation (IYS). The IYS will expose the seriousness of the global sanitation crisis and aim to accelerate progress for meeting the MDG target of halving, by 2015, the proportion of the world's population without sustainable access to basic sanitation. However, if trends since 1990 continue, the world is likely to miss the MDG target by almost 600 million people.

The Five Key Messages of the International Year of Sanitation

1. Sanitation is vital for human health. Poor sanitation and hygiene causes death and disease.
2. Sanitation generates economic benefits. Improved sanitation has positive impacts on economic growth and poverty reduction.
3. Sanitation contributes to dignity and social development. Sanitation enhances dignity, privacy and safety, especially for women and girls.
4. Sanitation helps the environment. Improved disposal of human waste protects the quality of drinking-water sources and improves community environments.
5. Improving sanitation is achievable. Working together, households, communities, governments, support agencies, civil society and the private sec-

tor have the resources, technologies and know-how to achieve the sanitation target.

World Water Week

The 2008 World Water Week in Stockholm is a conference devoted to discuss current progress and future prospects in the efforts to build a clean and healthy world. At the 2008 Water Week, special focus will be given to the challenge of the global sanitation crisis and the achievement of the Millennium Development Goal target on sanitation.

Another purpose of the 2008 World Water Week is to increase awareness of the downstream impacts of human activities. To reduce poverty and to meet an increasing demand for food, goods and services, intensive **exploitation** of natural resources will be necessary. When planning for new developments, consideration needs to be given to the effects of those developments and the increased waste that they carry to downstream bodies of water and aquatic ecosystems. An important goal of the 2008 Water Week is to find ways to integrate these complex issues of sanitation, water supply, ecosystem management and sustainable development into a single discussion.

Emergency Response Situations

In the aftermath of hurricanes, tsunamis, floods, earthquakes, or other disasters like war, one of the dangers is

Did You Know?

East, Southeast, and Western Asia, Northern Africa and Latin America and the Caribbean are on track to halve the proportion of people without basic sanitation by 2015. All other developing regions have made insufficient progress toward the MDG target. In sub-Saharan Africa, the absolute number of people without access to sanitation actually increased–from 335 million in 1990 to 440 million people by the end of 2004.

Water Supply & Sanitation Collaborative Council (WSSCC) and WASH

The WSSCC is an international organization that has worked since 1990 to provide adequate safe water supplies and sanitation for people around the world. One of the programs run by the WSSCC includes the Water supply, Sanitation and Hygiene (WASH) Coalitions. WASH coalitions raise awareness of water, sanitation, and hygiene issues.

always a lack of safe drinking water. UNICEF is working with the Norwegian government to provide water filtration systems to areas of the world that desperately need clean water, whether as the result of a flood or a drought. Ten units have been installed in Ethiopia since 2003, and similar units were used in Afghanistan, Mozambique, and the former Yugoslavia. The units consist of a tank with two hoses attached. Water is pumped up the hoses through filters and into a tank, where it is disinfected with chlorine. The safe, filtered water is then sent to large storage tanks. The systems are relatively small, easy to use, and work on almost every water source. If used properly they will run for ten years.

What Can YOU Do?

The most important thing you can do to help in the fight against water pollution is to get involved in protecting and preserving water! On an individual level that means you need to use less water and pollute as little as possible.

- Pick up debris you find lying in streams, lakes, or coastal waters, but be sure to wash your hands afterwards. DO NOT touch anything that appears to be medical waste—leave that for men and women in hazmat suits!

- Get involved with some of the programs listed in this chapter, or one of the many groups not covered here. There are many organizations working to provide safe water and sanitation to the world, or working to protect our coastal waters.

- Make your voice heard in the millennium goals project. Add your name to let your government know that you want the world leaders to honor their commitments to the MDG goals for water quality and sanitation. www.endpoverty2015.org/why-me

Be Responsible

You can do several things to help protect your watershed, water quality and coastal waters:

- *Use pesticides and fertilizers on your yard sparingly and correctly. Compost organic waste.*

- *Properly dispose of toxic substances like paint and paint thinners, automotive fluids, and cleaning products. Participate in "amnesty days" or take toxic wastes to appropriate collection sites.*

- *Curb your dog and properly dispose of pet waste. Do not leave it on the ground or throw it down a storm drain.*

- *Maintain your septic tank if you have one. Frequent pumping, proper drain field maintenance, and careful waste disposal will prolong the life of your system and prevent discharge of untreated sewage to ground and surface waters.*

- *Pick up litter when you see it and properly dispose of your own trash.*

- *Get involved in volunteer clean-up, monitoring, and environmental protection efforts. Possibilities range from helping with mailings and phone campaigns to stenciling storm drains and participating in beach and stream cleanups.*

- Send e-cards from the Water Supply & Sanitation Collaborative Council www.wsscc.org/en/e-cards/ index.htm to spread the word about the global sanitation crisis. Education and knowledge are the first steps to change. Your card may encourage someone to participate more fully in one of the MDG programs to help meet the sanitation goal for 2015.

STRAIGHT FROM THE SOURCE

From the Water Supply & Sanitation Collaborative Council document,
Nigeria Launches Hand Washing Campaign

First Lady, Hajia Turai Yara'dua on Tuesday May 20 2008 launched the National Hand Washing Campaign in Abuja, Nigeria. The event, which had in attendance top government officials, wives of government officials, members of Civil Society Organizations, stakeholders in the water and sanitation sector, media and school children, witnessed the symbolic hand washing by the wife to the President of the Federal Republic of Nigeria.

Speaking at the event, Hajia Yara'dua stressed the importance of hand washing in breaking the transmission of diseases. She said commitment to wash hands at critical moments can mark an end to many diseases like diarrhea, and cholera among others and expressed her commitment to supporting the promotion of the hand washing campaign as well as provision of clean water and sanitation in Nigeria. The First Lady thereafter performed the symbolic hand washing signaling the launch of the campaign.

Minister of Environment, Housing and Urban Development, Hajia Halima Tayo Alao in her address said the National Hand Washing campaign was part of the activities for the 2008 International Year of Sanitation. She said the campaign was a global initiative for promoting good hygiene practices as a strategy for improved public health.

She said: "the act of hand washing appears simple and often taken for granted, yet it is rated as the most important thing to do to prevent ill health. Many people do not practice the basic personal hygiene of washing the hands before cooking or serving food at homes/restaurants, or after using the toilets".

The Minister said the campaign will move to all the six geopolitical zones of the country in line with the third target of the national plan of action which is hygiene promotion.

She said the federal government has established the environmental health officers' registration council of Nigeria and the national environmental standards regulations enforcement agency in order to ensure proper sanitation across the country.

UNICEF Country Representative, Dr. Linlim Robert said that there are clear scientific evidence that support the practice of hand washing, stating that hand washing reduces diarrhea by 30%. He also noted that the prevalence of diarrhea in Nigeria is about 18% and that 60% of infant deaths under five are caused by diarrhea. He called on the Nigerian populace to adopt hand washing as a way of life and re-orient them through a collective effort.

What Do You Think?

- Do you believe that simply adopting hand washing could improve the public health of Nigeria?

- Do you think there are any other simple measures as basic as hand washing that could improve public health dramatically?

Find Out More

Gender and Water Alliance
www.genderandwater.org

Water Supply & Sanitation Collaborative Council
www.wsscc.org

World Water Week
www.worldwaterweek.org

United Nations. Millennium Development Goals Report. 2007.

For More Information on Health & the Environment

Books

Gordon, Bruce, Richard Mackay and Eva Rehfuess. *Inheriting the World: The Atlas of Children's Health and the Environment.* World Health Organization, 2004.

Ho, Mun S. and Chris P. Nielsen, eds. *Clearing the Air: the Health and Economic Damages of Air Pollution in China.* Cambridge, MA: MIT Press, 2007.

Kusinitz, Marc. *Poisons and Toxins.* New York: Chelsea House Publications, 1992.

MacDonald, John J. *Environments for Health.* New York: Earthscan Publications, 2006.

McCally, Michael, ed. *Life Support: The Environment and Human Health.* Cambridge, MA: MIT Press, 2002.

Nadakavukaren, Anne. *Our Global Environment: a Health Perspective.* 6th edition. New York: Waveland Press, 2005.

Nakaya, Andrea C. *Is Air Pollution a Serious Threat to Health?* New York: Greenhaven Press, 2004.

Netzley, Patricia D. *Contemporary Issues: Issues in the Environment.* New York: Lucent Books, 1997.

Vesley, Donald. Human *Health and the Environment: A Turn of the Century Perspective.* New York: Springer, 1999.

Web Sites

Air Pollution
health.nih.gov/result.asp/19

Air Quality
www.epa.gov/airnow/

CDC: Environmental Health
www.cdc.gov/Environmental/

EPA: Environmental Kids Club
www.epa.gov/kids/

The Green Squad
www.nrdc.org/greensquad/intro/intro_1.asp

Health and Environmental Linkages Initiative
www.who.int/heli/en/

International Year of Sanitation
www.who.int/water_sanitation_health/hygiene/iys/
about/en/index3.html

Kids for Saving Earth
www.kidsforsavingearth.org/index_low.html

Library of Congress Environmental; Photographs
memory.loc.gov/ammem/award97/icuhtml/aephome.html

Public Health and the Environment
www.who.int/phe/en/

Teen Ink
www.teenink.com/Environment/index.php

Toxic Household Cleaners
www.tutorials.com/08/0858/0858.asp

United Nations Population Fund
www.unfpa.org/

Water and Sanitation Quiz
www.unicef.org/voy/explore/wes/1883_wes_quiz.php

Glossary of Environmental Health–Related Terms

When you're reading about environmental health, especially in some of the more technical government reports, you may encounter many unfamiliar medical terms. This glossary can help you better understand the words scientists and other experts use when talking about the effects of environmental pollution on human health.

Absorption
The process of taking in; for a person or an animal, this refers to a substance getting into the body through the eyes, skin, stomach, intestines, or lungs. Chemicals can be absorbed into the bloodstream after breathing or swallowing. Chemicals can also be absorbed through the skin, into the bloodstream, and then transported to other organs. Not all chemicals breathed, swallowed, or touched are absorbed.

Acute
Occurring over a short time, usually a few minutes or hours. An acute exposure only lasts for up to 14 days; it can result in short-term or long-term health effects. An acute effect happens a short time after exposure.

Additive Effect
The body's response to exposure to multiple substances that equals the sum of responses of all the individual substances added together.

Adverse Health Effect
A change in body function or cell structure that might lead to disease or health problems.

Ambient
Surrounding. Ambient air usually means outdoor air (as opposed to indoor air).

Analyte

A chemical for which a sample (such as water, air, blood, urine, or another substance) is tested and measured in the laboratory. For example, if the analyte is mercury, the laboratory test will determine the amount of mercury in the sample.

Antagonistic Effect

A biologic response to exposure to multiple substances that is less than would be expected if the known effects of the individual substances were added together.

Aquatic Ecosystem

A community of organisms that live together in a body of water and are interdependent.

Aquifer

A geological formation where the spaces between rock particles, sand, or gravel are completely filled with water. Water pumped from aquifers is referred to as "groundwater".

Background Level

A typical or average level of a chemical in the environment. Background often refers to naturally occurring or uncontaminated levels. Background levels in one region of the world may be different than those in other areas.

Bedrock

The solid rock underneath surface soils.

Biodegradation

Decomposition or breakdown of a substance through the action of microorganisms (such as bacteria or fungi) or other natural, physical processes (such as sunlight).

Biologic Indicators of Exposure Study

A study that uses medical tests and other markers of exposure in human body fluids or tissues to confirm human exposure to a hazardous substance.

Biological Monitoring

Measuring chemicals, hormone levels, or other substances in biological materials (blood, urine, breath, or hair) as a measure of chemical exposure and health in humans or animals. A blood test for lead is an example of biological monitoring.

Biologic Uptake

The transfer of substances from the environment to plants, animals, and humans.

Biomedical Testing

Testing of persons to find out whether a change in a body function might have occurred because of exposure to a hazardous substance in the environment.

Biota

Plants and animals in an environment. Some of these plants and animals might be sources of food, clothing, or medicines for people.

Body Burden

The total amount of a chemical in the body. Some chemicals build up in the body because they are stored in body organs like fat or bone or are eliminated very slowly.

Cancer

Any one of a group of diseases that occur when cells in the body become abnormal and grow or multiply out of control.

Cancer Risk

The theoretical risk for getting cancer if exposed to a substance every day for 70 years (a lifetime exposure). The true risk might be lower.

Carcinogen

A substance that causes cancer.

Case Study
A medical evaluation of one person or a small group of people to gather information about specific health conditions and past exposures.

Case-Control Study
A study in which a group of people with a disease (cases) are compared to people without the disease (controls) to see if their past exposures to chemicals or other risk factors were different.

Central Nervous System (CNS)
The part of the nervous system that includes the brain and the spinal cord.

Chronic
Occurring over a long period of time, several weeks, months, or years.

Chronic Exposure
Contact with a substance that occurs over a long time (more than a year).

Cluster Investigation
A review of an unusual number, real or perceived, of health events (for example, reports of cancer) grouped together in time and location. Cluster investigations are designed to confirm case reports; determine whether they represent an unusual disease occurrence; and, if possible, explore possible causes and contributing environmental factors.

Cohort Study
A study in which a group of people with a past exposure to chemicals or other risk factors are followed over time and their disease experience compared to that of a group of people without the exposure.

Comparison Value (CV)

Calculated concentration of a substance in air, water, food, or soil that is unlikely to cause harmful (adverse) health effects in exposed people. The CV is used as a screening level during the public health assessment process. Substances found in amounts greater than their CVs might be selected for further evaluation in the public health assessment process.

Composite Sample

A sample which is made by combining samples from two or more locations. The sample can be of water, soil, or another substance found in the environment.

Concentration

The amount of one substance dissolved or contained in a given amount of another substance. For example, sea water has a higher concentration of salt than fresh water does.

Contaminant

Any substance found somewhere (for example, the environment, the human body, or food) where it is not normally found. Contaminants are usually referred to in a negative sense and include substances that spoil food, pollute the environment, or cause other adverse effects.

Delayed Health Effect

A disease or an injury that happens as a result of exposure that might have occurred in the past.

Dermal

Having to do with the skin. For example, dermal absorption means absorption through the skin.

Dermal Contact

Touching the skin.

Detection Limit

The smallest amount of substance that a laboratory test can reliably measure in a sample of air, water, soil, or other medium.

Dose

The amount of substance to which a person is exposed. Dose is a measurement of exposure and is often expressed as milligram (amount) per kilogram (a measure of body weight) per day (a measure of time) when people eat or drink contaminated water, food, or soil. In general, the greater the dose, the greater the likelihood of an effect. An "exposure dose" is how much of a substance is encountered in the environment. An "absorbed dose" is the amount of a substance that actually got into the body through the eyes, skin, stomach, intestines, or lungs. For radioactive chemicals, dose is the amount of energy from radiation that is actually absorbed by the body. This is not the same as the measurement of the amount of radiation in the environment.

Dose-Response Relationship

The relationship between the amount of exposure to a substance and the resulting changes in body function or health.

Environmental Media and Transport Mechanism

Environmental media include water, air, soil, plants, and animals. Transport mechanisms move contaminants from the source to points where human exposure can occur. The environmental media and transport mechanism is the second part of an exposure pathway.

EPA

United States Environmental Protection Agency.

Epidemiology

The study of the occurrence and causes of health effects in human populations. An epidemiological study often

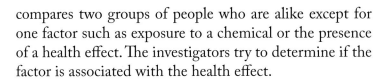

compares two groups of people who are alike except for one factor such as exposure to a chemical or the presence of a health effect. The investigators try to determine if the factor is associated with the health effect.

Exposure
Contact with a chemical by swallowing, breathing, or direct contact (such as through the skin or eyes). Exposure may be either short term (acute) or long term (chronic).

Exposure Assessment
The process of finding out how people come into contact with a hazardous substance, how often and for how long they were in contact with the substance, and how much of the substance they were in contact with.

Exposure-Dose Reconstruction
A method of estimating the amount of people's past exposure to hazardous substances. Computer and approximation methods are used when past information is limited, not available, or missing.

Exposure Investigation
The collection and analysis of information from an environmental site and biologic tests to determine whether people have been exposed to hazardous substances.

Exposure Pathway
The route a substance takes from its source (where it began) to its end point (where it ends), and how people can come into contact with (or get exposed to) it along the way. An exposure pathway has five parts: a source of contamination (such as an abandoned business); an environmental media and transport mechanism (such as movement through groundwater); a point of exposure (such as a private well); a route of exposure (eating, drinking, breathing, or touching), and a receptor population (people potentially or actually exposed). When all five parts are present, the exposure pathway is termed a completed exposure pathway.

Exposure Registry
A system of the ongoing follow-up of people who have had documented environmental exposures.

Feasibility Study (FS)
A study that compares different ways to clean up a contaminated site. The feasibility study recommends one or more actions to remediate the site.

Geographic Information System (GIS)
A mapping system that uses computers to collect, store, manipulate, analyze, and display data. For example, GIS can show the concentration of a contaminant within a community in relation to points of reference such as streets and homes.

Gradient
The change in a property over a certain distance. For example, lead can accumulate in surface soil near a road due to automobile exhaust. As you move away from the road, the amount of lead in the surface soil decreases. This change in the lead concentration with distance from the road is called a gradient.

Groundwater
Water beneath the earth's surface in aquifers (as opposed to surface water)

Half-Life
The time it takes for half the original amount of a substance to disappear. In the environment, the half-life is the time it takes for half the original amount of a substance to disappear when it is changed to another chemical by bacteria, fungi, sunlight, or other chemical processes. In the human body, the half-life is the time it takes for half the original amount of the substance to disappear, either by being changed to another substance or by leaving the body. In the case of radioactive material, the half life is the amount of time necessary for one half the initial number of radioactive atoms to change or transform into another

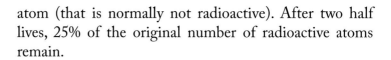

atom (that is normally not radioactive). After two half lives, 25% of the original number of radioactive atoms remain.

Hazard
A source of potential harm from past, current, or future exposures.

Hazardous Waste
Potentially harmful substances that have been released or discarded into the environment.

Health Assessment for Contaminated Sites
Determination of actual or possible health effects due to environmental contamination or exposure. It includes a health-based interpretation of all the information known about the situation. The information may come from site investigations (environmental sampling and studies), exposure assessments, risk assessments, biological monitoring, or health effects studies. The health assessment is used to advise people on how to prevent or reduce their exposures, to determine what action to take to improve the situation, or the need for additional studies.

Health Effects Studies (related to contaminants)
Studies of the health of people who may have been exposed to contaminants. They include, but are not limited to, epidemiological studies, reviews of the health status of people in exposure or disease registries, and doing medical tests.

Health Registry
A record of people exposed to a specific substance (such as a heavy metal), or having a specific health condition (such as cancer or a communicable disease).

Incidence
The number of new cases of disease in a defined population over a specific time period.

Ingestion

Swallowing (such as through eating or drinking). After ingestion, chemicals may be absorbed into the blood and distributed throughout the body.

Inhalation

Breathing. People can take in chemicals by breathing contaminated air.

Interim Remedial Measure (IRM)

An action taken at a contaminated site to reduce the chances of human or environmental exposure to site contaminants. Interim remedial measures are planned and carried out before comprehensive remedial studies. They can prevent additional damage during the study phase, but don't interfere in any way with the need to develop a complete remedial program. An example of an interim remedial measure is removing drums of chemicals to a storage facility from a site that has drums sitting in an empty field.

In Vitro

In an artificial environment outside a living organism or body. For example, some tests are done on cell cultures or slices of tissue grown in the laboratory, rather than on a living animal.

In Vivo

Within a living organism or body. For example, when scientific research is done on whole animals, such as rats or mice.

Latency period

The period of time between exposure to something that causes a disease and the onset of the health effect. Cancer caused by chemical exposure may have a latency period of 5 to 40 years.

Leaching
As water moves through soils or landfills, chemicals in the soil may dissolve in the water, thereby contaminating the groundwater. This is called leaching.

Maximum Contaminant Level (MCL)
The highest (maximum) level of a contaminant allowed to go uncorrected by a public water system under federal or state regulations. Depending on the contaminant, allowable levels might be calculated as an average over time or might be based on individual test results. Corrective steps are implemented if the MCL is exceeded.

Media
Elements of a surrounding environment that can be sampled for contamination: usually soil, water, or air. Plants as well as humans (when sampling body substances such as blood or urine) and animals (such as sampling fish to update fish consumption advisories) can also be considered media. The singular of "media" is "medium."

Metabolism
All the chemical reactions that enable the body to work. For example, food is metabolized (chemically changed) to supply the body with energy. Chemicals can be metabolized by the body and made either more or less harmful.

Metabolite
Any product of metabolism.

Morbidity
Illness or disease. A morbidity rate for a certain illness is the number of people with that illness divided by the number of people in the population from which the illnesses were counted.

Mortality
Death. Usually the cause (a specific disease, a condition, or an injury) is stated along with this term.

Mutagen
A substance that causes mutations (genetic damage).

Mutation
A change (damage) to the DNA, genes, or chromosomes of living organisms.

Odor Threshold
The lowest concentration of a chemical that can be smelled. Different chemicals have different odor thresholds. Also, some people can smell a chemical at lower concentrations than others can.

Organic
Generally considered as originating from plants or animals, and made primarily of carbon and hydrogen. Scientists use the term organic to mean those chemical compounds which are based on carbon.

Permeability
The property of permitting liquids or gases to pass through. A highly permeable soil, such as sand, allows a liquid to pass through quickly. Clay has a low permeability.

Persistence
The quality of remaining for a long period of time (such as in the environment or the body). Persistent chemicals (such as DDT and PCBs) are not easily broken down.

Plume
An area of chemicals moving away from its source in a long band or column. A plume, for example, can be a column of smoke from a chimney or chemicals moving with groundwater.

Point of Exposure
The place where someone can come into contact with a substance present in the environment (see **Exposure Pathway**).

Population
A group or number of people living within a specified area or sharing similar characteristics (such as occupation or age).

Prevalence
The number of existing disease cases in a defined population during a specific time period.

Prevention
Actions that reduce exposure or other risks, keep people from getting sick, or keep disease from getting worse.

Protocol
The detailed plan for conducting a scientific procedure. A protocol for measuring a chemical in soil, water, or air describes the way in which samples should be collected and analyzed.

Radioisotope
An unstable or radioactive isotope of an element that can change into another element by giving off radiation.

Radionuclide
Any radioactive isotope of any element.

Receptor population
People who could come into contact with hazardous substance.

Registry
A systematic collection of information on persons exposed to a specific substance or having specific diseases.

Remedial Investigation (RI)
An in-depth study (including sampling of air, soil, water, and waste) of a contaminated site needing remediation to determine the nature and extent of contamination. The remedial investigation (RI) is usually combined with a feasibility study (FS).

Remediation

Correction or improvement of a problem, such as work that is done to clean up or stop the release of chemicals from a contaminated site. After investigation of a site, remedial work may include removing soil and/or drums, capping the site, or collecting and treating the contaminated fluids.

Risk

Risk is the possibility of injury, disease, or death. For example, for a person who has measles, the risk of death is one in one million.

Risk Assessment

A process which estimates the likelihood that exposed people may have health effects. The four steps of a risk assessment are: hazard identification (Can this substance damage health?); dose-response assessment (What dose causes what effect?); exposure assessment (How and how much do people come into contact with it?); and risk characterization (combining the other three steps to characterize risk and describe the limitations and uncertainties).

Risk Management (or Reduction)

The process of deciding how and to what extent to reduce or eliminate risk factors by considering the risk assessment, engineering factors (Can procedures or equipment do the job? For how long and how well?), social, economic, and political concerns.

Route of Exposure

The way in which a person may contact a chemical substance. For example, drinking (ingestion) and bathing (skin contact) are two different routes of exposure to contaminants that may be found in water. See **Exposure**.

Safe

Free from harm or risk. Exposure to a chemical usually has some risk associated with it, although the risk may

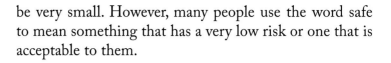

be very small. However, many people use the word safe to mean something that has a very low risk or one that is acceptable to them.

Sample
A portion or piece of a whole. A selected subset of a population or subset of whatever is being studied. For example, in a study of people the sample is a number of people chosen from a larger population. (See **Population**.) An environmental sample (for example, a small amount of soil or water) might be collected to measure contamination in the environment at a specific location.

Sample Size
The number of units chosen from a population or an environment.

Solubility
The largest amount of a substance that can be dissolved in a given amount of a liquid, usually water. For a highly water-soluble compound, such as table salt, a lot can dissolve in water. Motor oil is only slightly soluble in water.

Solvent
A liquid capable of dissolving or dispersing another substance (for example, acetone or mineral spirits).

Source of Contamination
The place where a hazardous substance comes from, such as a landfill, waste pond, incinerator, storage tank, or drum. A source of contamination is the first part of an **Exposure Pathway**.

Special Populations
People who might be more sensitive or susceptible to exposure to hazardous substances because of factors such as age, occupation, sex, or behaviors (for example, cigarette smoking). Children, pregnant women, and older people are often considered special populations.

Stakeholder
A person, group, or community who has an interest in activities at a hazardous waste site.

Statistics
A branch of mathematics that deals with collecting, reviewing, summarizing, and interpreting data or information. Statistics are used to determine whether differences between study groups are meaningful.

Superfund
The United States' federal and state program that investigates and cleans up inactive, hazardous waste sites.

Surface Water
Water on the surface of the earth, such as in lakes, rivers, streams, ponds, and springs.

Synergistic effect
A biologic response to multiple substances where one substance worsens the effect of another substance. The combined effect of the substances acting together is greater than the sum of the effects of the substances acting by themselves.

Target Organ
An organ (such as the liver or kidney) that is specifically affected by a toxic chemical.

Teratogen
A substance that causes defects in development between conception and birth.

Toxic Agent
Chemical or physical (for example, radiation, heat, cold, microwaves) agents that, under certain circumstances of exposure, can cause harmful effects to living organisms.

Toxicology
The study of the harmful effects of substances on humans or animals.

Tumor
An abnormal mass of tissue that results from excessive cell division that is uncontrolled and progressive. Tumors perform no useful body function. Tumors can be either benign (not cancer) or malignant (cancer).

Volatile
Evaporating readily at normal temperatures and pressures. The air concentration of a highly volatile chemical can increase quickly in a closed room.

Volatile Organic Compound (VOC)
An organic chemical that evaporates readily. Petroleum products such as kerosene, gasoline, and mineral spirits contain VOCs. Chlorinated solvents, such as those used by dry cleaners or contained in paint strippers, are also VOCs.

Bibliography

Bernard, Susan M., Jonathan M. Samet, Anne Grambsch, Kristie L. Ebi, and Isabel Romieu. "The Potential Impacts of Climate Variability and Change on Air Pollution-Related Health Effects in the United States," *Environmental Health Perspectives* 109, supp. 2 (May 2001).

Ebi, Kristie, Nancy Lewis, and Carlos Corvalan. "Climate Variability and Change and Their Potential Effects on Small Island States," *Environmental Health Perspectives* 114, no. 12 (December 2006): 1957-1963.

European Union, "EUROPA-Activities of the European Union on Energy": http://europa.eu/pol/ener/index_en.htm (accessed June 6, 2008).

Frumkin, Howard. "Climate Change, the Public Health Response," *The American Journal of Public Health* 98, no. 3 (March 2008).

Hales, Simon, Simon Lewis, Tania Slater, Julian Crane, and Neil Pearce. "Prevalence of Adult Asthma Symptoms in Relation to Climate in New Zealand," *Environmental Health Perspectives* 106, no. 9 (September 1998): 607-610.

Jepma, Catrinus J., and Mohan Munasinghe. *Climate Change Policy: Facts, Issues, and Analyses.* Cambridge, UK: Cambridge University Press, 1998.

Johansen, Bruce E. *The Global Warming Desk Reference.* Westport, CT: Greenwood Press, 2001.

Kovats, R. S., D. H. Campbell-Lendrum, A. J. McMichael A. Woodward, and J. S. Cox. Early Effects of Climate Change: Do They Include Changes in Vector-Borne Disease?" *Philosophical Transactions: Biological Sciences,* 356, no. 1411 (July 29, 2001).

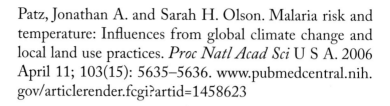

Patz, Jonathan A. and Sarah H. Olson. Malaria risk and temperature: Influences from global climate change and local land use practices. *Proc Natl Acad Sci* U S A. 2006 April 11; 103(15): 5635–5636. www.pubmedcentral.nih.gov/articlerender.fcgi?artid=1458623

Schneider, Stephen H, and Terry L. Root, eds. *Wildlife Responses to Climate Change: North American Case Studies.* Washington, DC: Island Press, 2002.

Shiquang, Wan, Yuan Tong, Sarah Bowdish, Linda Wallace, Scott D. Russell, and Yiqi Luo. "Response of an Allergenic Species, *Ambrosia psilotachya,* to Experimental Warming and Clipping: Implications for Public Health," *American Journal of Botany.* 89, no. 11 (November 2002).

Tibbetts, John. "Driven to Extremes: Health Effects of Climate Change," *Environmental Health Perspectives* 115, no. 4 (April 2007): A196-A203.

United Nations Framework on Climate Change, "The Kyoto Protocol": http://unfccc.int/kyoto_protocol/items/2830.php (accessed June 6 2008).

Vidal, John. "In the Land Where Life Is On Hold," *The Guardian* (June 30, 2005).

Weart, Spencer R. *The Discovery of Global Warming.* Cambridge, MA: Harvard University Press, 2003.

World Health Organization European Office, "Euro-Heat: Improving Public Health Responses to Heat Extremes." www.euro.who.int/eprise/main/who/progs/gch/Topics/20050524_2#F1 (accessed June 5, 2008).

World Health Organization. Fighting Malaria: Stories From Two Villages www.who.int/features/2005/malaria/en/index.html (accessed June 24, 2008)

World Health Organization. Living a Normal Life with Asthma www.who.int/features/2007/asthma/en/index.html (accessed June 24, 2008)

Index

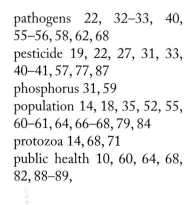

Picture Credits

CDC: pp. 28, 47, 48, 54, 56, 59, 67, 74
Carr, Janice: p. 71
Farmer, Charles N: p. 69
Healy, Dr. George: p. 72
Hayes, Dr. R.O.: p. 40

Dreamstime
  Icholakov: p. 39
  Idrutu: p. 10

khwi: p.16
lorna: p. 26
les3photo8: p. 13
Riekefoto: p. 18
shaileshnanal p. 15
Spepple22: p. 42
travismanley: p. 45

To the best knowledge of the publisher, all other images are in the public domain. If any image has been inadvertently uncredited, please notify Harding House Publishing Service, Vestal, New York 13850, so that rectification can be made for future printings.

About the Author

Cordelia Strange is an anthropologist by training and a naturalist at heart. She has a lifelong interest in education and environmental preservation. She lives in upstate New York with her husband and an orange cat. This is her first book for AlphaHouse.

About the Consultant

Elise DeVore Berlan, MD, MPH, FAAP, is a faculty member of the Division of Adolescent Health at Nationwide Children's Hospital and an Assistant Professor of Clinical Pediatrics at The Ohio State University College of Medicine. She completed her Fellowship in Adolescent Medicine at Children's Hospital Boston and obtained a Master's Degree in Public Health at the Harvard School of Public Health. Dr. Berlan completed her residency in pediatrics at the Children's Hospital of Philadelphia, where she also served an additional year as Chief Resident. She received her medical degree from the University of Iowa College of Medicine. Dr. Berlan is board certified in Pediatrics and board eligible in Adolescent Medicine. She provides primary care and consultative services in the area of Young Women's Health, including gynecological problems, concerns about puberty, reproductive health services, and reproductive endocrine disorders.

Anne Nadakavukaren is the author *Our Global Environment: A Health Perspective.* She has taught at Illinois State University, and she also served on Illinois's Structural Pest Control Advisory Council, an advisory group to the Department of Public Health. She is currently a member of the Illinois Low-Level Radioactive Waste Advisory Taskforce.